POW!

Pierre

+ Henriette

Henriette Piché

Printed in Canada by Apex Graphics Ltd.

ISBN 0-9735032-0-3

Especially for my children

Daniel
Valérie
Rodrigue
Pierre

but also for all who have known and appreciated Pierre.

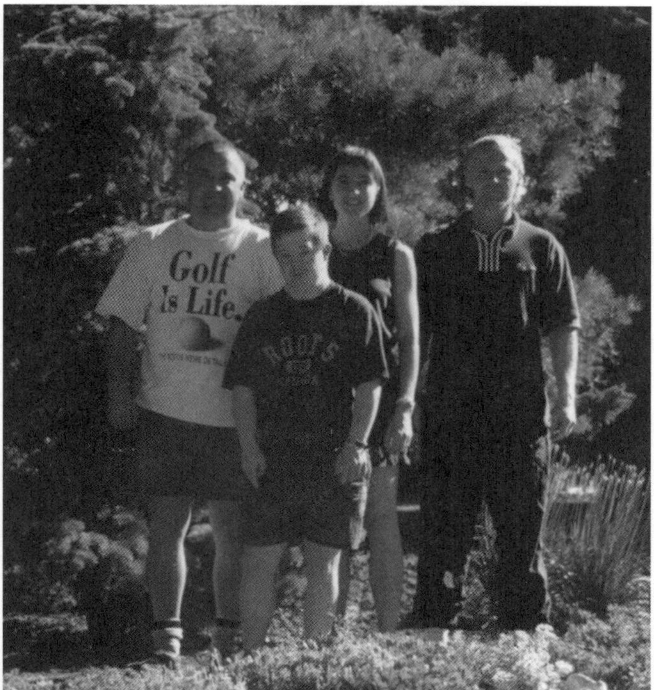

Table of Contents

Prologue...vii

I Birth 1
II Decision... 7
III Life Gets Better 13
IV Another Hero 17
V School 21
VI Puberty Crisis/Depression............. 37
VII IPI 43
VIII Medicine Hat................................. 53

Epilogue... 61

Testimonials 65

Prologue

Pierre was our fourth child born in five years. I was 26 years old when he was born. In the sixties, much stigma was attached to being retarded and the normal thing to do was to 'place' such a child. Reasons given: A handicapped child requires a lot of attention and time, therefore 'normal' kids as well as a marriage may suffer.

I write this book for my family and as a therapeutic challenge for myself. I hope it may even be helpful to other families who have chosen to have a 'special' child in their lives.

In italics I communicate Pierre's thoughts. Verbal expression is not his 'forte'; he communicates through his eyes and through his actions. As his mother I feel I can read his thoughts, feelings . . .

My name is Pierre. I have chosen my parents, Gilles and Henriette Fontaine-Piché. My older siblings are Daniel, Valérie and Rodrigue, five, three and two years of age respectively. I want to look different and be a challenge in life. My birth date is August 18, 1968. I'm a Down syndrome.

I
Birth

Mother's Perspective

I am so looking forward to giving birth to this fourth child. Last night I dreamt that it is a girl and she's dark like Rodrigue. Her name is Barbara. Now that I'm awake the name just doesn't sound right in French–too many 'r's'. It would be nice to have a little sister for Valérie. Daniel prefers a little brother. Even though I get sicker with each pregnancy, I enjoy motherhood and my dream of having six children in as many years makes sense to me. I grew up in a family where the age difference between me and my siblings is four, eight and fourteen years. I feel I missed out because we were all so far apart. Gilles' seven siblings are all close in age, and it is so much fun to listen to their 'growing up' stories. Therefore, it's important to me that my children be close in age so they can enjoy each other's company.

At last: signs of the impending arrival by the newest little Piché.

"How come it is not an easier birth than this?" I think to myself. It should be a breeze after Rod's nearly pleasant birth only two years ago. He finally arrives–at 2:25 a.m.– the 18th of August.

I'm so exhausted. I just need a little nap before I can hold my new son to my heart's content. Early morning I wake up and ask the nurse to bring him in so I can meet this new little person. Gilles is there too. We both comment on how he's not too pretty.

"You know, Gilles," I reassure him, " it's no wonder he's so misshapen after what he went through–look at his fat right cheek and flat nose; such tiny little eyes, kind of slanted, but then *pépère* Fontaine, my grandfather, had small eyes; one ear is turned like a small cabbage leaf. His hair is reddish like Daniel's. Well, even though he's not the prettiest child, he'll fill out eventually and look better." Gilles seems to be listening as he examines his new son.

"So, what do you think we should name this one?" I ask. "So far I've named the boys and you've named the girl. Remember, I always wanted to call our first daughter Désirée, but you preferred Valérie so you said, 'OK, let's settle this by putting the two names in a hat, and whichever one you pick is what she will be called.' Well, to this day, I'm pretty sure that hat contained two Valéries."

Gilles, laughing, said, "I guess you'll never know because you never checked!"

"I'd like to name him Pierre," I said. "You know how much I admire Pierre Elliot Trudeau, and there doesn't seem to be many Pierres on either side of the family."

Gilles agrees this is a good name and it is also the name of the first Piché to set foot on Canadian soil in the latter part of the 1600s.

Further examination by both of us reveals that Pierre has the right amount of toes and fingers. I wonder out loud, "How come his colouring is so purple? And his feet are so flaky dry! I'll have to ask the doctor." Gilles leaves for work.

The doctor comes in later that morning and I tell him what I've noticed about Pierre. He doesn't say much. "Hey," I tell him, "I'm so happy it is all over. It was such a tough delivery. And I'm ready to go home. I've got Mom to help me and I should really be home with the rest of them."

Doc replies, "We'll see how things go. How soon you get your strength back."

Three days later it's great to be home with the whole crew. Thank goodness for Mom. Every morning she is there to help me bathe and feed the kids. Pierre is such a good baby.

"Sometimes I think he knows he has to wait his turn," I tell Mom. "But I wonder why I feel there is such a black cloud hanging over this house?"

She replies, "You're probably just tired as this is such a very busy household."

"You know, Mom, sometimes he seems to stop breathing. I run to the crib, touch him and the breathing returns to normal. I check him often–just in case."

Time goes by so quickly and Mom is right–four kids five years and under–this house is really busy. Soon already it's the first week of October, and Gilles tells me, "The doctor is coming tonight because you haven't been to his office for the six-week check up. He wants to see how you and Pierre are doing."

"Great," I reply. "Saves me the hassle of making an appointment and going there." Doc arrives around seven. "So how are things?" he asks.

"Fine," I reply. "I just worry a little about Pierre's sometimes 'irregular' breathing."

"Go and get him so I can check him over," says Doc. As I hand Pierre over to him he says: "Have you noticed how his tongue is protruding?" Doc turned him around. "Do you see how his neck is shaped? How flat the back of his head is? How small his ears are and that they're lower than they should be?" He then takes Pierre's little hand in his and says, "I want to show you the crease in his right hand. Did you notice his short stubby fingers?"

I look as he points out these various imperfections and he continues, "He has very wide spaces between his toes and you'll notice that his skin is different. We call that mottled skin."

Now I am very afraid; I interrupt and ask, "What does this mean?"

Doc answered, "He's what you call a mongoloid. In other words, he's retarded and this can range from mild to severe. At the moment there's no sign of heart problems or lung problems, but that can also be part of his makeup."

I'm crying inside and outside. Doc continues, "Because of your three other children, I think the best place for Pierre is in an institution where he will get the best of attention. A retarded child needs a lot of care and it could be very difficult on your other children because you may not have enough time for them."

I tell him, "But he's no trouble. He is such a good

baby; he never cries and already he sleeps through the night!"

Doc leaves.

My mother and Alain, Gilles' brother and a priest with the OMIs, walk in. Major hugs are exchanged. I can't stop crying.

Gilles tells me, "For a while I've been noticing that every now and then Pierre has this certain look that doesn't seem right. Remember when Brigitte (our sister-in-law, a Registered Nurse) kept Pierre for a day? She picked up right away that Pierre is mongoloid. She called Alain and described Pierre's mongoloid traits. They were sure we didn't know. Alain came to see me the next morning at work and confirmed what I have been noticing. I went to see Doc and he also validated that Pierre has a problem. I asked Doc to come and tell you tonight."

Mom then spoke up, "Jo Anne (my 13-year-old sister) noticed it the first week you were out of the hospital. She told me, "Pierre looks like Margo" (a child with Down syndrome, five years older than Pierre).

I felt disbelief at all I was hearing.

Mom continued, "I went to see the doctor and he confirmed that Pierre is retarded. I also asked if he could wait until you were a little stronger before telling you."

Gilles said, "Doc also mentioned that two other babies born about the same time as Pierre are suspected of being like him, but the parents may not know yet. The other two doctors that delivered those babies have no conclusive evidence they are mongoloid."

I feel like I'm having an out-of-body experience.

The subject comes up again that Pierre must be 'put away'. Alain names institutions in Manitoba where Pierre can be accommodated. I tell them, "It will kill me to put him away." I cuddle Pierre as he nestles nicely in my neck. How can I possibly let this child go? I need to look at his face. His little slanted eyes are wide open and all of a sudden his little hand stretches out and takes my necklace in his hand. I laugh and cry at the same time.

It will kill me to put him away.

Pierre's perspective

I am loved. I will survive.

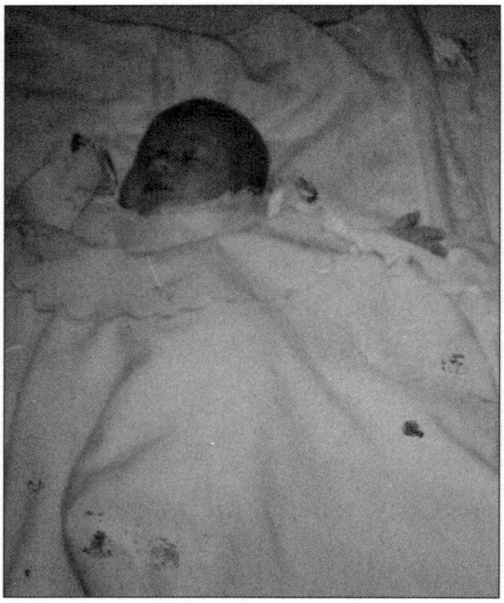

Baptismal Day

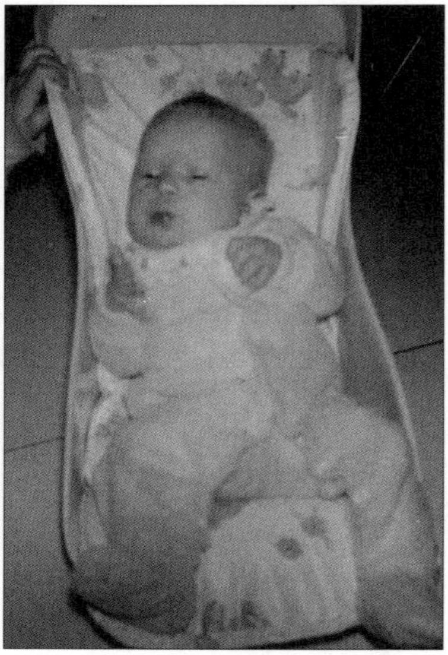

Pierre is about one month

II

Age 6 weeks to 11 months
Decision

Mother's Perspective

Sleep is impossible. Pierre is in our bed, between us. I keep checking him out. I am unable to comprehend what is happening. I just can't discuss that this child has to be put away. It doesn't make sense. We leave that touchy subject for later.

Finally, morning rolls around. Gilles leaves for work. Mom comes in to help with the daily ritual. What a sad morning. My neighbour, Bev, pops in for coffee. She is the first one to whom I verbalize what has taken place in the last twelve hours. All three of us are crying. In the afternoon I visit the doctor; I need something to settle me down and, of course, more discussion about Pierre takes place. He gives me tranquilizers.

"Why me?" I keep asking myself.

I hold this baby in my arms as often as I can–how can I ever let him go? How destructive will it be if this baby goes and I'm only half a mother to the other three?

Within the month Mom and Dad keep all four while Gilles and I make the hour-and-a-half trip to visit the Moose Jaw Training School–an institution for retarded people. We take a tour of the facility. It is worse than awful. How can anyone leave a baby in such a place? He will die and so will I.

At the end of the tour we meet the doctor in charge of the establishment. He declares that the facility does not take babies anymore; instead, a support system exists through the Saskatchewan Association for the Mentally Retarded (SAMR). He gives us the address in Saskatoon and explains that the Association can help us guide Pierre through as normal a life as possible. There is a God! And He is there for Pierre and/or for me.

"That's it!" I tell myself, as we leave the Training School. "I don't need these tranquilizers any more." They are garbaged and traded in for pen and paper. I write to Mr. John Dolan, c/o SAMR in Saskatoon, asking for

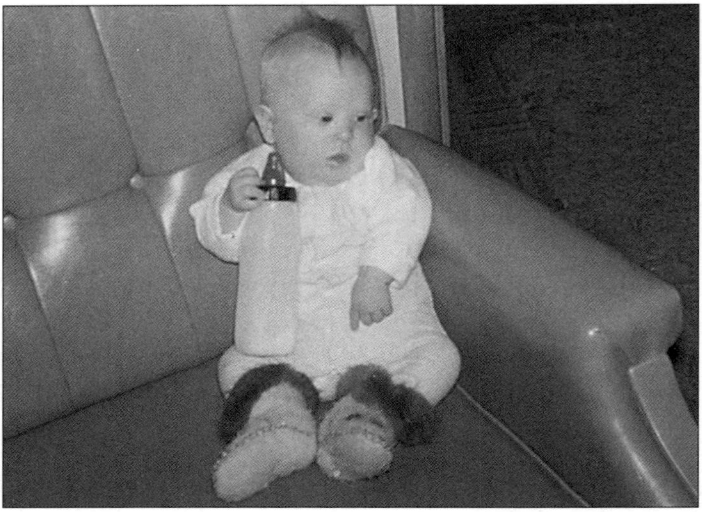

Age 11 months

information. He comes to our house and explains what Pierre's future could be like i.e. walking, toileting, schooling–he may be educable, meaning that he may thrive in a school environment or trainable, meaning that he may be only able to learn some lifeskills. Books and pamphlets are left for us to study. Mr. Dolan advises of the advantages of belonging to the SAMR.

After searching in Gravelbourg and area, five other couples with children with challenges are invited to our home to discuss what we have learned from Mr. Dolan. How interesting that, within five years, three children with Down's have been born in Gravelbourg. That night, in 1968, the Gravelbourg Branch of the SAMR is created.

Social workers become part of our lives to be a support for Pierre as well as for us as parents. As the Social Worker checks Pierre's body he gives us assurance that Pierre's legs are strong and that he should walk way before the standard four or five years. Toilet training may take six to eight years.

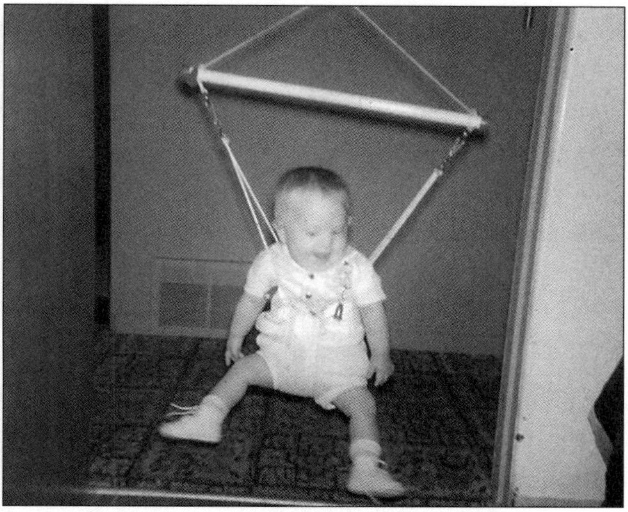

Jolly Jumper is part of exercise

As far as schooling is concerned, there are not that many options in a small community.

Daily exercises become very important to strengthen arms, legs, and torso. There's a lot of activity to keep Pierre awake and make him aware of his surroundings. The other three are encouraged to play their games around him and have him hold things for them. The daily hustle and bustle operation becomes a cooperative effort by the whole family.

Whenever we are out I notice how people react to Pierre. It hurts me when they glance at him and then quickly look away.

At one point, all six of us travel to Regina to see a speech therapist. As parents we are concerned that plans to educate the older three in French could cause problems for Pierre in our bilingual community of thirteen hundred people. The speech therapist assures us that having to deal with two languages will not be harmful and that Pierre may eventually speak both.

At eleven months–July 1969–Pierre becomes very ill. He is dehydrated due to nausea and diarrhea. The doctor admits Pierre to the Gravelbourg Hospital and after two days Pierre becomes a patient at the Regina General Hospital. He is totally lifeless. While in the Regina emergency, I talk softly in his ear and hold him close for the four hours it takes to get a bed. At one point during those four hours he grabs hold of my hair. I'm so grateful he is showing signs of life.

Being on an intravenous for a couple of days, his body is able to mend itself. Three weeks later, he can sit up by himself. Progress is happening!

Pierre's perspective

I am loved. I am cared for. I will survive.

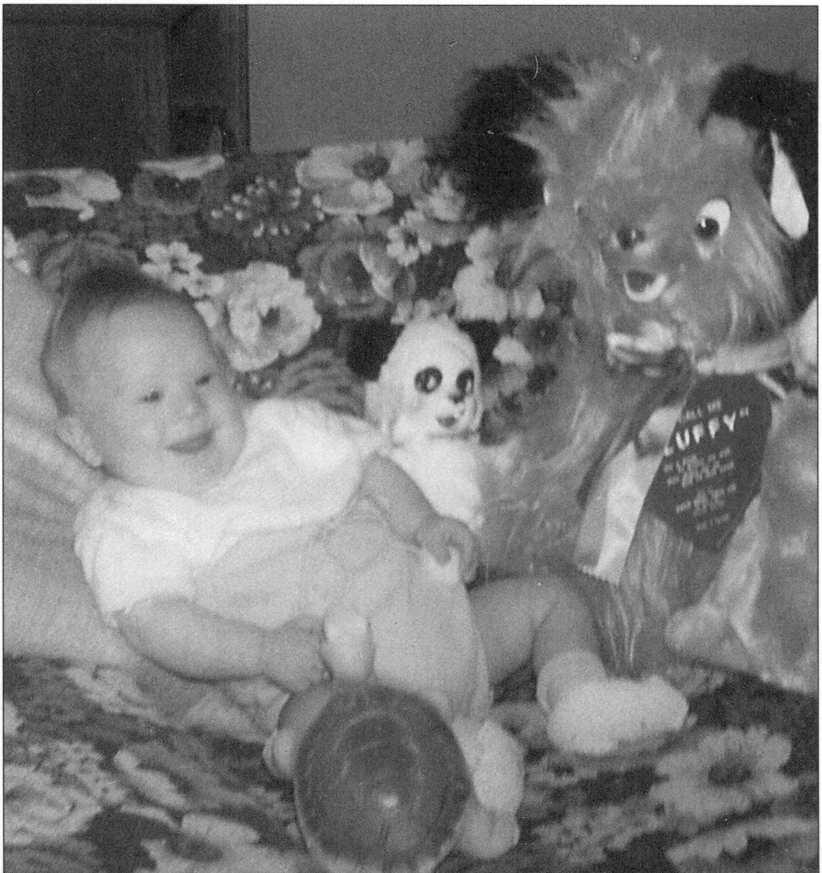

III

Age to 1 – 2 1969–1970

Life Gets Better

Mother's perspective

The daily exercises continue. Now that Pierre sits without help, he reaches for things that are around him and tastes all of them. He can maneuver a spoon so he eats by himself. Learning to crawl now becomes priority. It is not easy. He still has not mastered getting from his tummy to the sitting position in order to go forth on all fours.

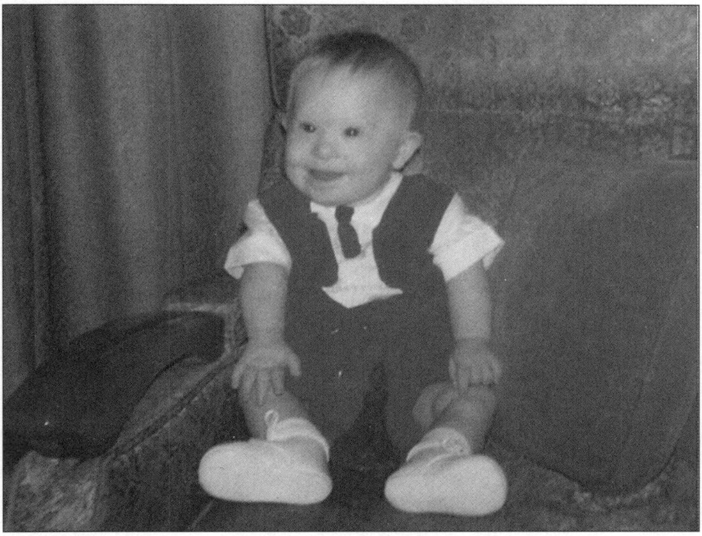

Gilles' playtime with Pierre includes holding Pierre in the palm of his hand and making him dance. Pierre sits tall and straight and holds Gilles' finger for support. Gilles sings a neat little medley as he keeps time with the music. Pierre totally loves it.

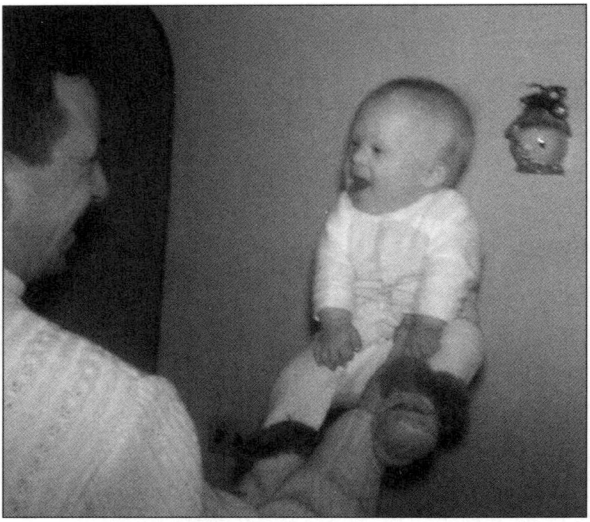

Gilles making Pierre dance

Although Pierre is still young, a topic of conversation that keeps coming up is the eventuality of his educational needs. Through our SAMR meetings, it is obvious that there is a need for a classroom for kids like Pierre in Gravelbourg. We ask Alain to help us draw up a brief which we present at a meeting comprised of officials from the Gravelbourg School Board, Saskatchewan Government, as well as our Social Worker and the parents. The meeting concludes with a decision that the Gravelbourg School Board is willing to open a special class for the handicapped as long as there are seven students. Only one more student is required to fill the quota and the Social Worker promises that the Moose Jaw Training School can provide that student as long as he/she has an approved home to live in. Pierre's future is assured. So we think!

Life continues in the Piché household. Pierre is getting very close to his two years. Finally he is crawling–on his stomach but not on all fours. Part of the morning routine for Pierre and me, while the older children are at Kindergarten and school, is to go for coffee at Mom's. Pierre sits in the crook of my dad's arms. He is still very small–the size of a nine-month-old at best. As Pierre is not overly active he and Dad, who suffers from emphysema and asthma, make a good team. It's a good thing, too, for Pierre gets to spend a lot of time with his grandparents because of the involvement of his siblings in hockey, figure skating, ballet.

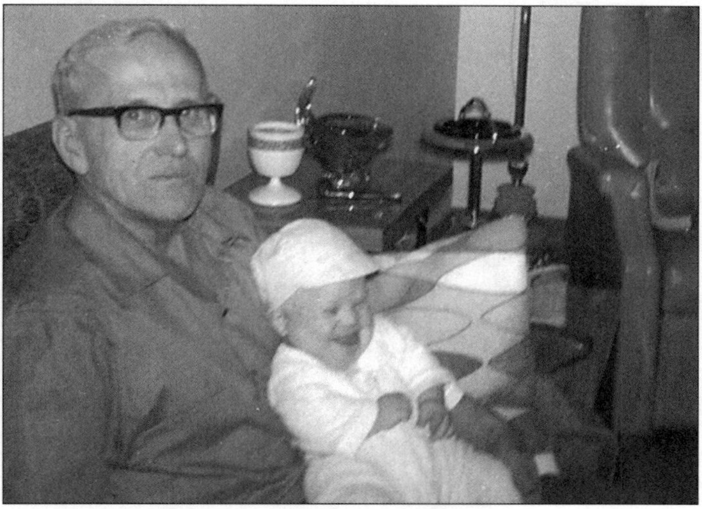

Pierre and Père Fontaine

It is interesting to watch him perform one of his habits. He extends his left arm out to the left side as far as it will go–slowly moving it to the right–watching his fingers. At one point, he loses sight of his hand, then refocuses on it when it comes back into his view. He can do this for a long time, over and over. Another one of his habits is to hold and feel hair between his thumb and index finger while he sucks his tongue. It can be his own hair or anyone else's.

I feel peace and quiet within myself. Life is so much better. Now if we can only get that schooling off the ground.

Pierre's perspective

I like to watch . . . Dan plays with blue and red soldiers. He makes them fight one against the other. He asks me to choose which colour. Val and Rod usually play around me especially when I'm in my 'jolly jumper'.

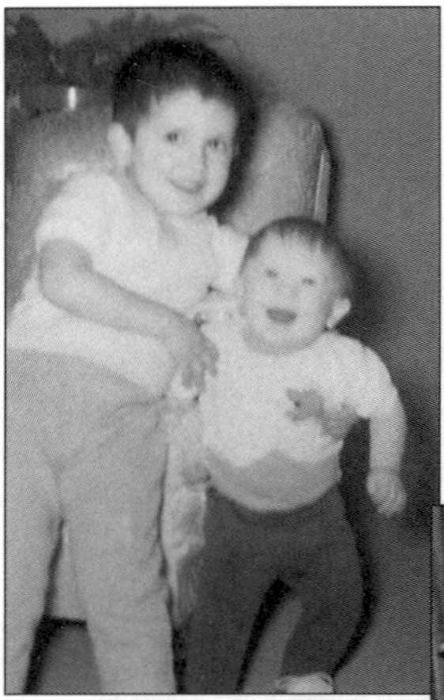

Rod trying to show Pierre how to walk

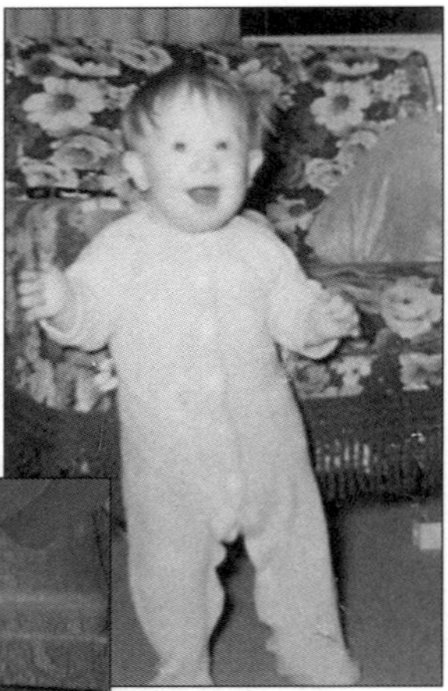

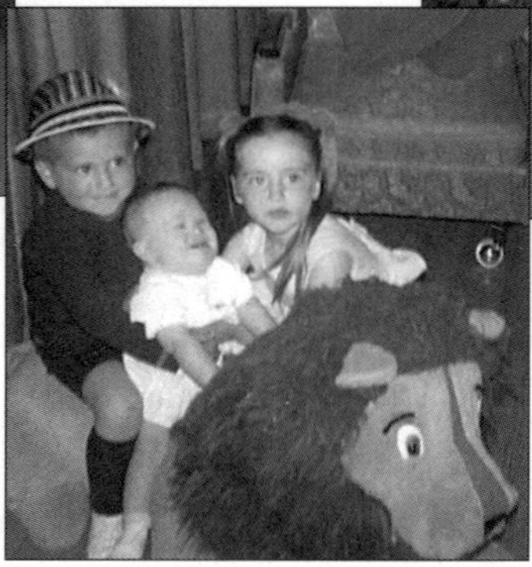

IV

Age 2 – 3   1970–1972
Another Hero

Mother's perspective

It is August 18, 1970, and a big celebration is happening for Pierre's second birthday. He crawls to the bathroom, still on his stomach, and says: "uh, uh, uh" to let

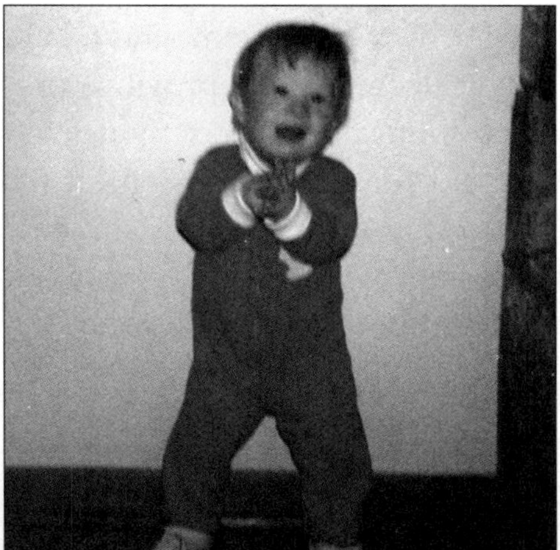

Walking at last – 2 years, 1 week

us know he needs to use the facility. I am so proud of him. Imagine being toilet trained before he can walk! Imagine defying the predictions of the professionals and the books!

A week after his second birthday, he leaves the security of my arms and walks, unaided, to Gilles. Jubilation. Busily exploring his environment at this new height he quickly gets into mischief. I love it.

The subject of Pierre's schooling and the promise of an extra student is always at the forefront of our minds. The process is just not progressing as fast as I would like it. In February of 1971, I receive a phone call from government officials advising they cannot provide an extra student. After two years of 'blood, sweat and tears' we're back to square one. Gilles is very angry.

Gilles makes an unannounced trip to see the manager of the Training School, where the Social Worker who promised us an extra student is employed. It proves fruitless. We are both frustrated.

However, in 1971, a New Democratic Party (NDP) government is newly elected in the province of Saskatchewan. Gravelbourg and district votes in a young, enthusiastic, Member of Legislative Assembly (MLA) by the name of Reg Gross. After cups of coffee, much conversation, and a file folder holding two years of paper work, Reg sets off to his new post and becomes my new hero.

It doesn't take long before a student is transferred from the Moose Jaw Training School to Gravelbourg. Thanks to Reg we now have seven students. The Gravelbourg School Board hires a teacher by the name of Vera Silzer. Pierre, at three years of age, attends school for an hour every morning.

After that major upheaval, our lives are back on track. By September, 1971, the four kids are where they should be. I'm happy.

Pierre's perspective

The chocolate cake is set before me so I can blow out the two candles. I need help–my siblings do that. I get that good stuff all over my face.

Walking is fun. I love to follow my brothers and sister.

V

Age 3–13   1971–1981

School

Mother's Perspective

Pierre can now say a few words, especially names of the people involved in his life. *Père* are his Grandfathers Piché and Fontaine, *Mère* is his Grandmother Fontaine, *Pom* is his Grandmother Piché, Gilles is *Jin*, I am *Mamaman*. His siblings are *Naniel, Bididi* and *Dig*. My sister JoAnne is

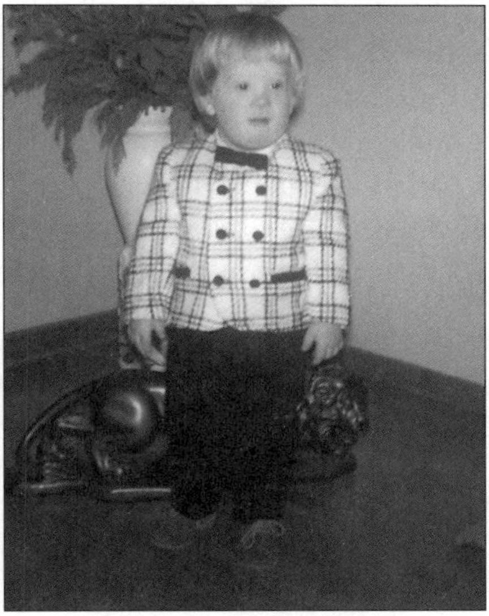

Pierre Piché, 3–4 years old

Shoshoi, and his teacher is *Silzer.* He is so cute in his size two jeans which he calls *gree.* Excuse me is *gildi.*

I don't know if he pronounces these names/words because that is what he hears or because that is the way they come out. His tongue is still too big and he always has to be reminded to remove his thumb from his mouth. Actually, a callous has formed on his thumb from this bad habit of chewing on it.

In the mornings I work as 'undersecretary' to the secretary of the school board, and, therefore it is *Père* Fontaine's duty to pick Pierre up after his hour at school. After Christmas Dad gets very sick and is hospitalized. I make arrangements with Silzer to keep Pierre for an extra half-hour until *Père* Piché can pick up Pierre. From that day on he attends school for an hour-and-a-half even though *Père* Fontaine is back on duty.

My sister, Alice (Pierre calls her *Calice*) and her husband, Guy, who live in Regina, often visit at Mom's with their two children, Guylaine and Gratien. Pierre ignores Guylaine, but is quite taken with Gratien. As soon as Gratien can walk, Pierre walks directly behind him, step for step. In the beginning Gratien is fearful of Pierre and keeps running to his mother. Eventually he learns to ignore Pierre, and Pierre finally gets over following him so closely.

Life is very busy with all the kids in various activities. Of course, Pierre doesn't fit into the pattern we have set for the other three, i.e., figure skating, hockey, ballet, piano. At age four and five we try him in figure skating, but he can't keep up. I'm disappointed a little bit, but it's OK.

Pierre's sporting talents are soon discovered to be running and jumping. He is a perfect candidate for Special

Olympics. There are many willing coaches including his teacher, Vera, as well as his Aunt JoAnne and his siblings.

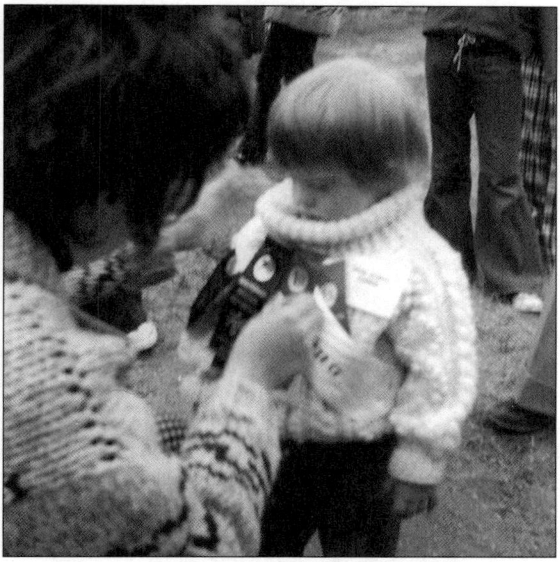

First Olympics

His first Olympics are held in Assiniboia and I quote from the June 7, 1973, *Gravelbourg Star*: " Four-year-old Pierre Piché received great applause throughout the day and achieved a total of 22 points." Size is probably what makes him interesting to watch; he still wears size two clothes. Every year brings in more red ribbons. To be truthful, he is sometimes alone in his category, and when he does have competition, he tends to wait for the competition to catch up. There's always a crowd urging him to get to the finish line.

Our seventh student from the Moose Jaw Training School does not work out. Each year, we have a meeting with the Gravelbourg School Board; I always feel threatened that the class will close because we don't have the magic

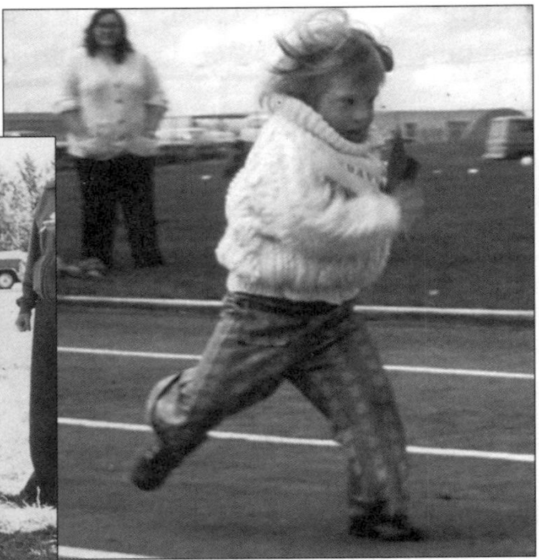

Running for Special Olympics

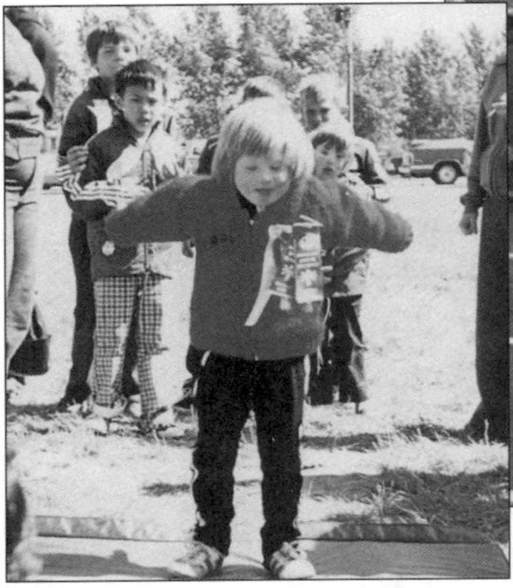

Standing broad jump

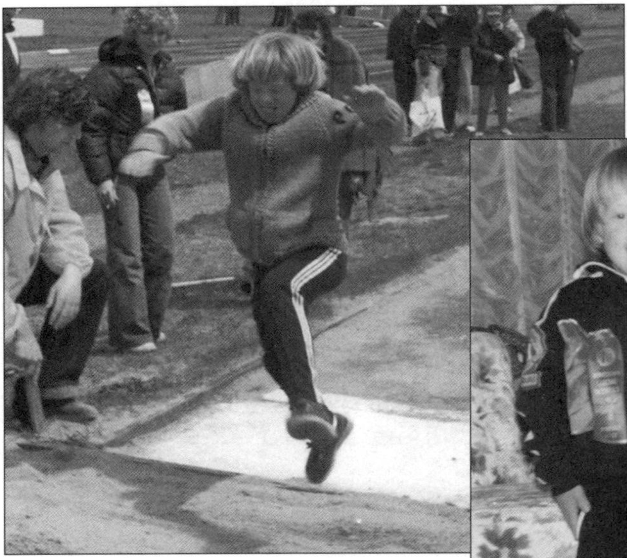

Running broad jump

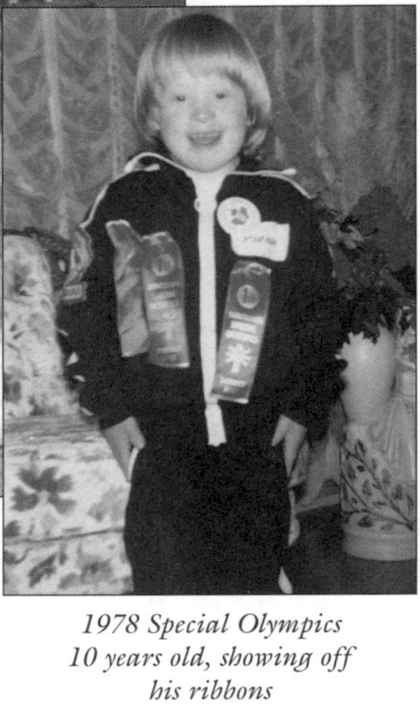

1978 Special Olympics
10 years old, showing off
his ribbons

number of seven students. The Board pays for the teacher, provides the classroom, and minimal supplies.

As the SAMR, Gravelbourg Branch, we raise funds for whatever materials Vera requires. We need more equipment to train for Special Olympics, more school supplies, more materials for crafts. We need money. We have a few tea and bake sales. That's OK, but surely there are better ways to raise more money, and more quickly! One day I decide to take a major plunge and as luck would have it, I fall into my element. I start organizing Fashion Shows. Everybody must model sewn, crocheted or knitted outfits. My friend, Leona, always ready to back me up in whatever schemes, provides the background music. Mother's Day is always the day picked for the show. And with so many people creating such beautiful things, why not have a raffle? I ask for donations of crafts.

Five days prior to the show I make an arrangement with the principal and ask grades four to seven students to

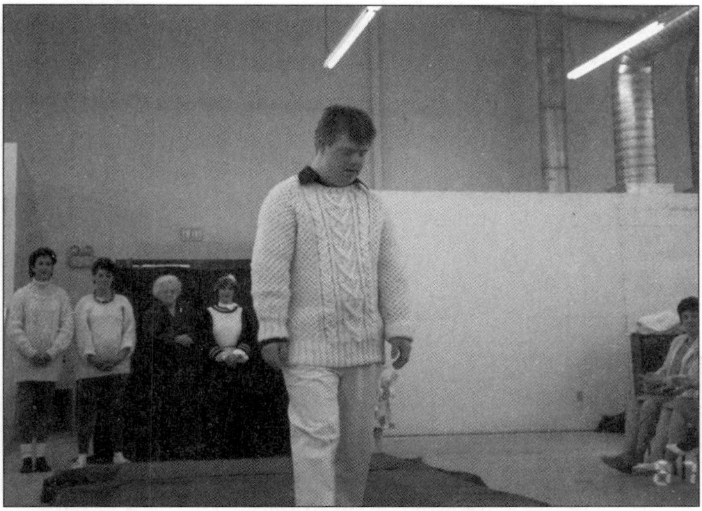

1987 Fashion Show

go on a three-day blitz to sell raffle tickets on the donated crafts. The first year generates $350 from the sale of raffle tickets and the fashion show entry fee; by the eleventh year sales are over $1000. Happiness is bliss!

Mère is an excellent knitter. The whole family gets new sweaters or outfits every year. *Mère's* fingers are very busy and, we, her daughters are always coming up with creative ideas for ourselves and our children!

To keep the audience entertained in between the fashions, Vera puts on a sport demonstration by the students–jumping, gymnastic bars, exercises on mats. The kids are fabulous. Every year this gets more involved and more entertaining.

What great support we get from the community of Gravelbourg and area! Models and spectators come from as far away as Mankota and Assiniboia, Coderre and Courval. Over the years there are many repeat seamstresses, crocheters and knitters, and always new participants.

So far we have not taken many trips as a family. In the summer of 1974, we decide to travel to Hay River, NWT, to visit Gilles' brother, Camille, with a stop over in Edmonton at Gilles' sister, Denise. This Aunt has a pool and it is Pierre's first encounter with swimming. He wears newly purchased wings and loves the water. On our return from Hay River, a week later, Pierre hardly needs his wings to navigate the water. He's a natural.

Now at age six–wearing size four–Pierre attends school all day. The SAMR Gravelbourg Branch request that our 'special class' students attend recess with the 'normal' kids. Sure, a few problems arise, but on the whole it's a very positive experience. I maintain that the more exposure Pierre has with normal kids, the better he will be–not to mention that it is also good for them to interact with handicapped ones.

A few more words are added to his vocabulary: *Pesaille* for chips, *Co-Coke* for Coke, *gummy* for dummy.

Part of Pierre's morning ritual is to join Gilles and me in bed–becoming the ham in the sandwich. One Christmas holiday he looks at us and says: "Silzer, pow!" as he gives his bum a slap. Vera always comes for supper before our monthly SAMR meetings so I tell her the story. She explains that Pierre is repeatedly pitching things up in the air, so one time she has resorted to a slap on his bum to make him stop. I imagine at times it must be frustrating dealing with all these different personalities. My point, however, is that Pierre can communicate even though his vocabulary is minimal.

Every summer, after lunch, from the age of ten, Pierre can be seen riding his bike on the streets of Gravelbourg heading towards the pool. Of course, the water wings were long ago discarded. Lifeguards are on duty and I trust God to have Traffic Angels on duty as well. Pierre has four stop signs to cross–which he doesn't obey until he's in the middle of the street. I get phone calls from concerned, irate, citizens telling me they nearly ran over Pierre. I reply, " I know he does not respect traffic and probably never will, but I also don't believe in locking him up in the yard. Should something happen we will cope with it knowing that Pierre would no doubt be at fault."

Gravelbourg is a close-knit community–everyone knows everyone else–a great place to raise a child like Pierre where he can have freedom of movement. As frightening as it is for those who nearly collide with him, I also know that those 1300 people look out for him. In one of his most brazen adventures he was riding his bike on the street heading towards the highway. A concerned citizen made him turn around and told him to go home. We always found out about his little excursions.

Honourable visitor

Saskatchewan's Lieutenant Governor is coming to visit Gravelbourg. The Special Class is honoured by being chosen to serve tea to His Excellency. Pierre is usually very well-mannered. However, on this particular afternoon Pierre decides to grace the elite entourage with one mega burp. Without skipping a beat, and before I had time to apologize, His Excellency, the Lieutenant Governor, says to Pierre, "Well, young man, that was very well brought up!" I was very appreciative of the diplomacy of this very kind gentleman.

The Plane

Gilles' sister, Terry, and husband, Aimé, live in Ferland, in south west Saskatchewan. They own a plane. Pierre loves planes and Aimé often gives Pierre rides. One time when Terry and Aimé are visiting, Terry says to Pierre, "Would you like to come to Ferland?" Pierre disappears. Five

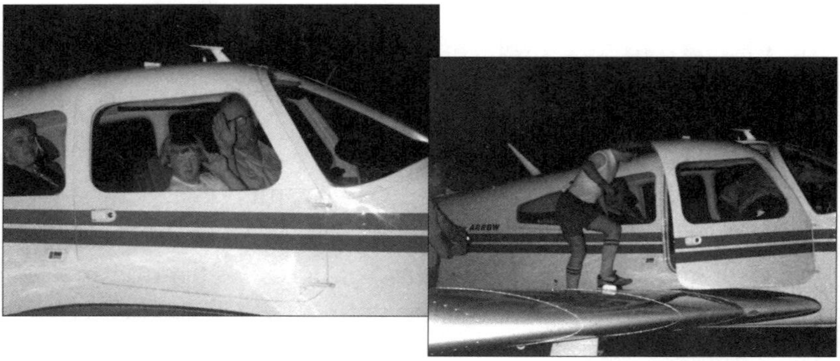

minutes later he comes up with a bag full of clothes ready for the trip. He's all smiles as he climbs aboard the plane. He stayed overnight and Gilles and I went to pick him up the next day.

Integration

The school board approaches the SAMR, Gravelbourg Branch, at one point, asking us to agree to an arrangement whereby Vera does remedial work with other students while ours attend regular classes from 1:00 until 2:15. What a fantastic arrangement! We discover that Pierre is hamming it up in class and is quite disruptive–the more the students laugh, the more he acts up. Gilles and I meet with the teacher and ask that she put her foot down, assuring her that he must be disciplined. She worries her regular students will think she is being 'mean' to Pierre. We insist that this is a good move for the special class and nothing must hinder its progress. As far as I know, since our meeting, Pierre is behaving.

The Wedding

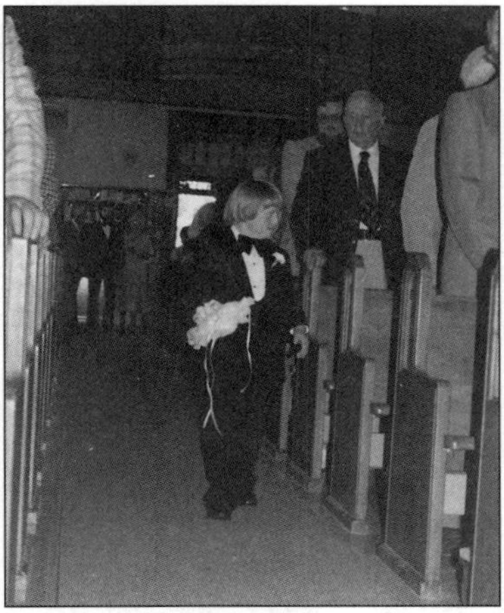

The Wedding

July 21, 1979, Pierre is ring bearer for JoAnne and John's wedding. At the rehearsal he uses the cushion as a baseball. He's still in the pitching-in-the-air phase! We are all a little nervous when the ceremony starts but he does it beautifully and keeps in step with his cousin, Guylaine, who is flower girl. He's pretty cute in his black tux. He's graduated to wearing a size six.

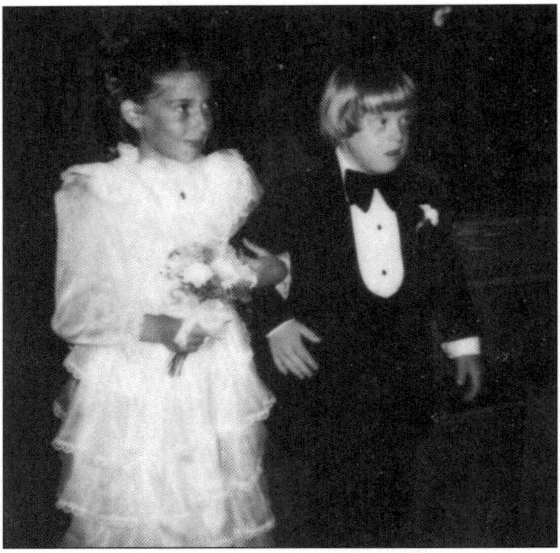

Guylaine & Pierre

Life Experience

Pierre loses his grandfather Piché the day before his eleventh birthday on August 17, 1979. His first encounter with death. I'm not sure if it is the loss of his grandfather or the amount of people in the house, but all of a sudden he is crying. I feel he needs to escape to a room where we can be just the two of us. We sit quietly and cuddle as I try to explain what is going on. As the days and weeks pass, he does not mention his grandfather.

Testing

In September 1979, Pierre is psychologically assessed as a nearly four-year-old academically and a seven-year-old socially.

Disneyland

Disneyland becomes a reality in October 1979. A lot of firsts for the kids: the 'big' plane ride–California–

Universal Studio–the Hulk–Knotts Berry Farm. But for Pierre, it is Goofy, Minnie, and his favourite Mickey Mouse–*Picky Pess* (a new word in his vocabulary). He sees them, runs after them, and they never refuse a reciprocated

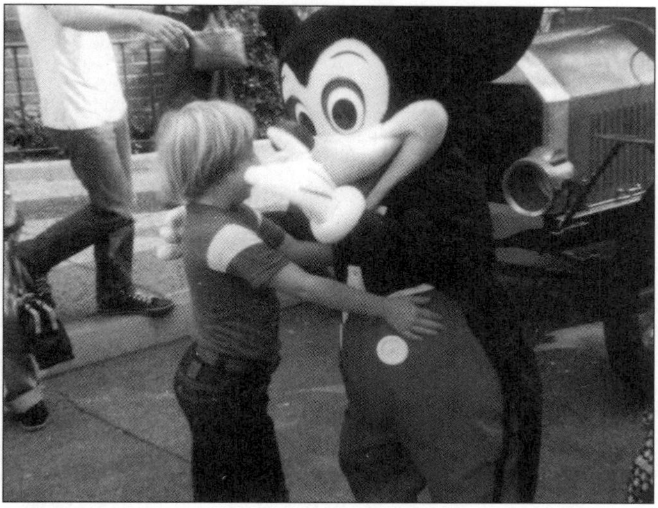

Pierre and "Picky Pess"

hug. What a great trip! Only one scary moment–we all get off the bus commenting on our tour of the day and we realize that Pierre has stayed on the bus. The alert driver sees us all running behind the bus and stops to let Pierre off. New rule–Gilles or I must remain behind Pierre at all times.

Another Life Experience

In May 1980, my dad ends up in the hospital for thirteen months. Pierre often goes on his bike to visit with him. They hold hands. I hear through the nurses that management at the hospital try to convince Pierre not to park his bike in the middle of the sidewalk. Also, he should refrain from using the elevator and take the stairs. But Pierre has a mind of his own! His bike retains its usual parking space, and when he feels no one is watching, he uses the elevator, sometimes in conspiracy with the nurses. *Père* Fontaine dies June 30, 1981. Pierre is nearly thirteen.

I try to explain, "Pierre, *Père* is gone up to heaven to see *Jésus*, just like *Père* Piché, and that is good." Long ago, I learned that it is best to keep messages short, and to the point, when speaking to Pierre. Shortly after, Pierre and I bike to the cemetery. Mom, my sister, Alice, and her son, Côme, who is five years old, are also visiting. Pierre says to Côme, "*Père en haut*" as his finger points to heaven. Côme, the realist, answers, "*Non,non, père en bas*!" as he points to the grave. A valid argument.

After eleven years, Vera Silzer decides she would like to take a different challenge and teach a regular class. Good work, Vera. We learned many things together.

A new teacher is hired for September 1982. Pat Préfontaine comes with new ideas and new projects. However, Gilles and I face a new challenge.

Pierre's Perspective

I like Gratien. He is smaller than me.

I love the chute for dirty clothes. I throw red cups down and see them break. I run to Mamaman and say, "Pow, pow, pow."

Everybody says, "Get your thumb out of your mouth." I always forget.

I'm very lucky to have Naniel, Bididi, Dig, that each take a week to walk to and from school with me. I forget about traffic! After I am six I go by myself.

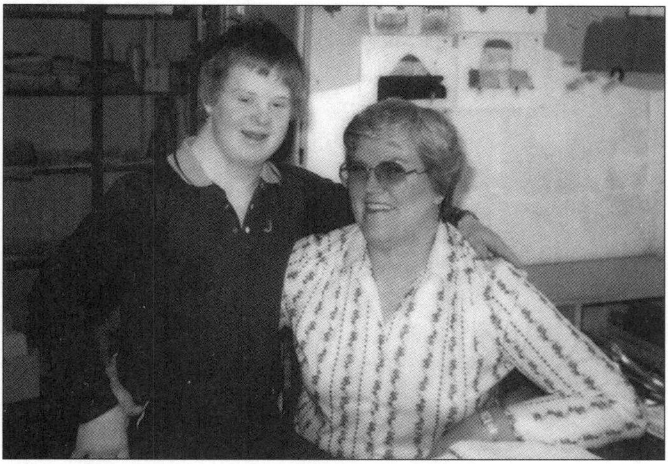

Pierre and Silzer

I learn to colour, do puzzles, with Silzer. I hate scissors, maybe it's because I am left-handed. I count to ten. I can name some colours. I read the Red, Yellow and Blue books of Dick and Jane. I have a box full of words on cards that I must practise every day. I hate that. She teaches me to 'pee' standing up. I can barely reach the rim and it's cold. We both giggle. Best part of the day is after school when I stop for my treat at Mère's. I get pesaille and Co-Coke and big hugs from Père and Mère. Then I run home across the back alley and ride my cousin Paul's little red pedal-car. I'm supposed to ride it only on the sidewalk, but I go on the street. Well, it is a car! RCMP stop me, "Get back on the sidewalk." I say: "oui" and move over. He leaves. I'm back on the street. Well, it is a car! My brothers tell Mamaman and I know she means business because she's pointing her finger at me. I forget and I'm on the street again.

One time at the Fashion Show I decide as I walk up the runway that I will try to scare the people–I do a quick action step. They laugh. I love it. They clap. I bow. The fun part of the show is when Silzer makes us do exercises on the stage. I love the applause. I like to bow.

I also play street hockey with Naniel and Dig and
all the other kids. I like that.

I'm 10 years old and now I ride my bike with no training wheels.
The first time I go around the block to show Père and Mère
that I have no more training wheels the neighbours
come out and cheer me on.

I skateboard too. I forget to watch for traffic. The skateboard,
with me on it, goes under this truck that is backing up. A man
runs to tell Mamaman. "Pow!" I tell her as she examines me.
No damage. The truck never knew I was under it.

The 'Dukes of Hazard' are on TV every week day.
No matter what I am doing I must watch them. I'm never late.

A place called 'The Arcade' opens on Main Street. One Saturday night,
I get on my bike and go there. Nice, noisy machines! A lot of
action. Oops! Here comes Mamaman. We get home
at the same time. She takes off my shoes. She knows I don't like
to walk without them! There's that finger again!

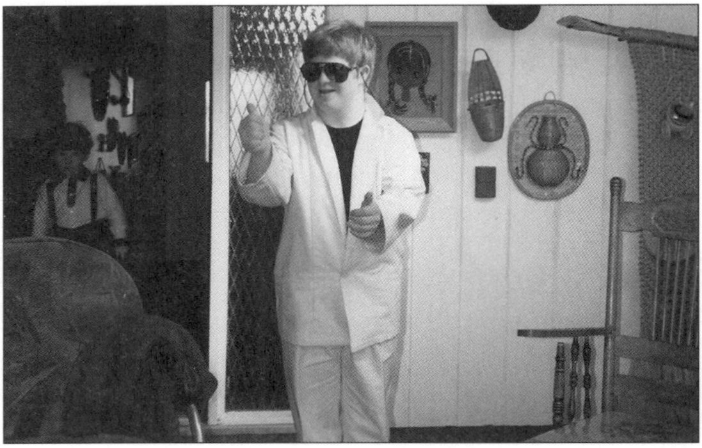

"The Fonz"

I like 'The Fonz'. He's a hero. I like to put glasses on and pretend I am him.

Bididi is my other mamaman. I know she's always there to help me and gives me lots of hugs. Dig is my friend. He plays with me. He lets me use his gloves, as long as I don't get them dirty. I borrow his hockey shoulder pads

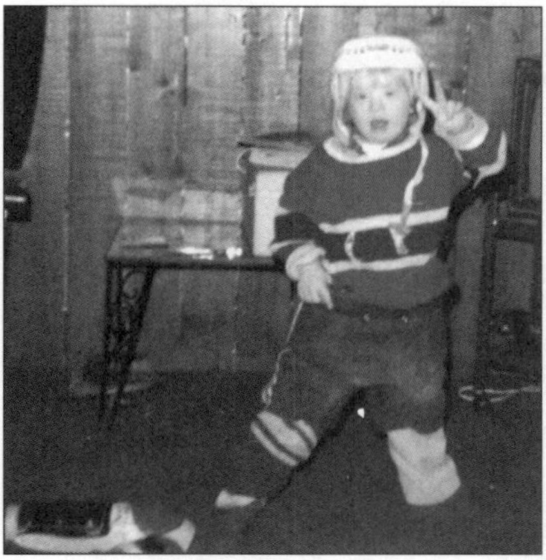

Borrowing Rod's equipment

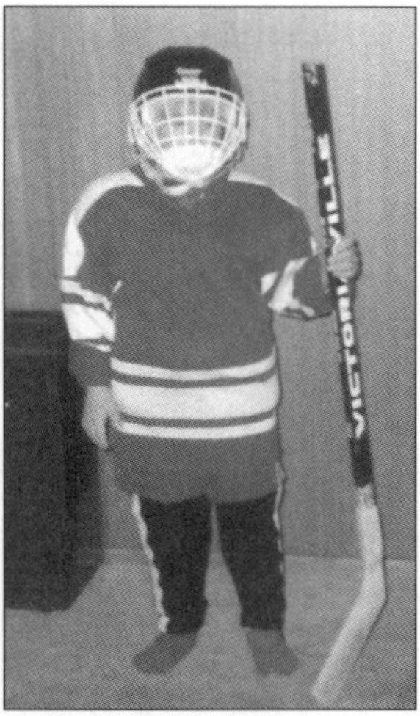

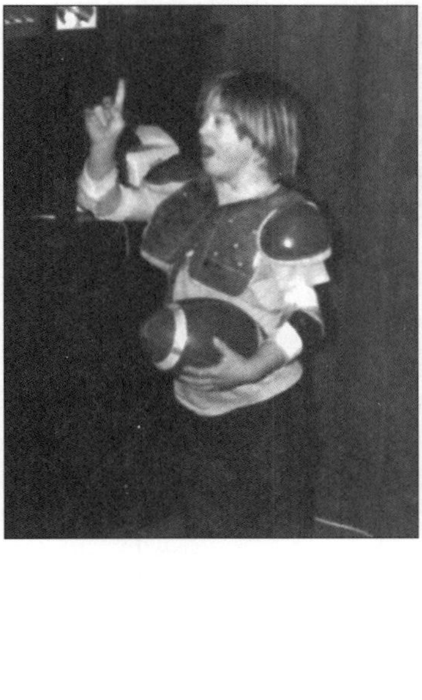

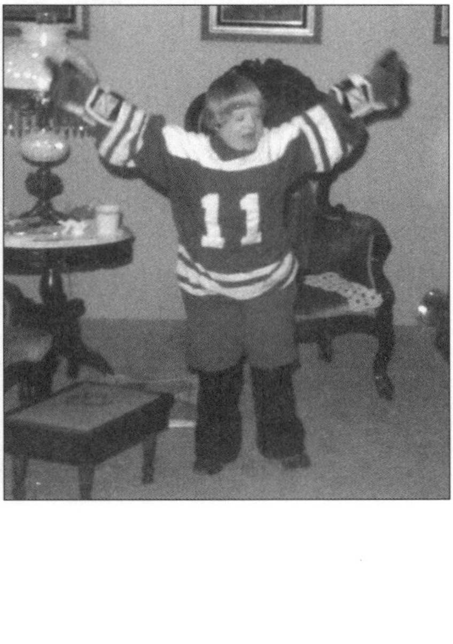

and his hockey sweaters, and it's OK. When Naniel passes by me he taps me on the head and says, "Hi, old chap."

Mère asks me to choose something out of the catalogue. I show her Chubakka. I love Chubakka. At Christmas I open a box and there he is. My Chubakka. I love Chubakka.

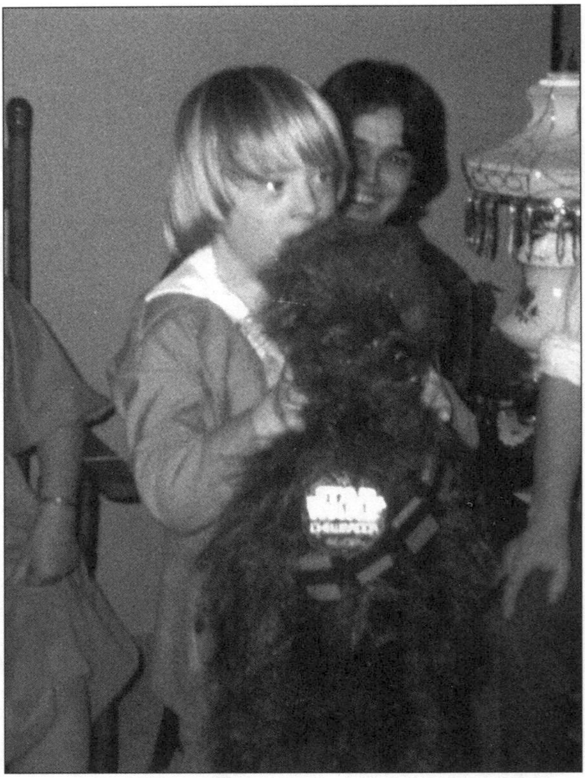

Chubakka

VI

Age 13 - 19 1982–1987

Puberty Crisis/Depression

Mother's Perspective

At age 14, Pierre is given three psychological tests in October of 1982: the Peabody Picture Vocabulary Test, the Vineland Social Maturity Scale and the Stanford-Binet Intelligence Test Form LM. This time, the results indicate his mental age at two years, eight months; his language age at two years, one month and his social scale at four years, four months. There has been no growth in Pierre's abilities since he was tested in 1979. He is regressing.

I don't know why this is happening. I do not feel in control of Pierre's situation. There is more thumb chewing. More twisting of his hair. His eyes don't express joy. Lots of giggling for no reason. At times he becomes very withdrawn. He does not seem interested in what goes on around him.

The first term report by Pat Préfontaine in November 1982, states that Pierre is adapting well to her as his new teacher and he is co-operative and pleasant to work with. Half the day is spent on academic activities and the other half on manipulative activities. Silzer is still part of his life as he goes to her while Pat works with remedial students.

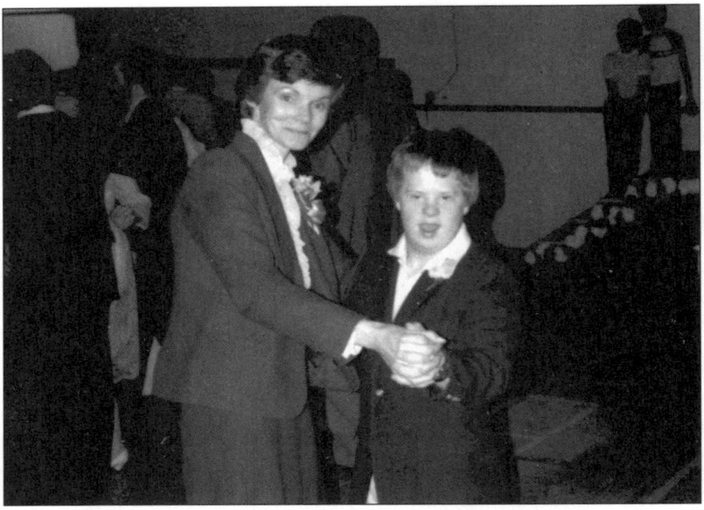

Pat and Pierre

Pat is innovative in trying to keep him occupied and happy during school hours. The end of June report in 1983 states that he has had a good year–can count to thirteen. She even has him repeating short phrases.

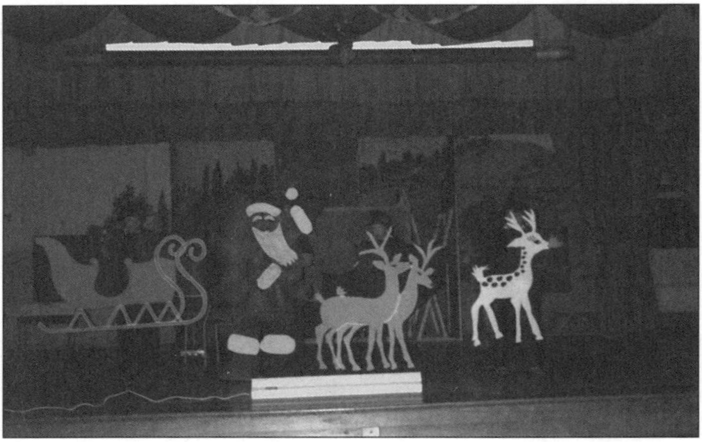

Black Art Theatre

In my mind the purpose of the fashion shows has always been two-fold; it is not only to bring in money, but also it is important for the community to see and accept those with mental challenges who also have a place in this world. When Pat takes over from Silzer in 1982, she introduces Black Art Theatre as part of the fashion show. What a beautiful concept and what a lot of work she puts into her creations. The kids do wonderfully well with it. Her efforts are very much appreciated by the audience.

Finally in October 1983, we get to see a specialist at the Alvin Buckwold Centre in Saskatoon. Pierre was having one of his 'typical' off-kind of day. The doctor's report reads: " . . . Pierre was obviously not relating to things around him but seemed to be in a world of his own, grinning vaguely and giggling from time to time. He still responds to his parents and cooperates when his attention can be focused for a short time."

Gilles and I are both disappointed. There is no definite answer. It comes down to one of three possible problems: chronic depression (but as he also has happy moods, it may be difficult for him to come out of it), atypical seizures, or the early beginning of Alzheimer's. An appointment is made to check for seizures. Amitriptyline is prescribed as an antidepressant. If it is Alzheimer's disease, there is nothing to do. How very discouraging.

The results in November from an EEG at the Valley View Centre show no signs of seizure activity. Thank God for that. Only two more possibilities to deal with, and those will take time and lots of patience.

Pat's end of the 1983 school year report states: "Pierre is bouncing back. And with his health improvement has come a renewed interest in life around him. He is starting to interact with his environment again."

It's got to be a depression that we are dealing with. I can cope better with that than the beginnings of Alzheimer's. At least then there may be a light at the end of the tunnel. The pills have stopped the giggling and night roving, so he does sleep better.

It is so difficult to see Pierre this way. During the past two summers he has not wanted to go swimming. It is hard to get him motivated. Thumb chewing and hair twisting is very exhausting to stop and so unpleasant for him because we keep after him. We discover the reason he is not interested in going outside is due to the antidepressant and the effect it has when one is in the sun. With the doctor's approval, we take him off the Amitriptyline. It can't get worse. However, even after weeks of not being on the drug, Pierre still doesn't venture outside or do much on his own.

The first term report of November 1984, reveals that Pierre is coping fairly well with a new schedule: mornings spent in the Special Class at the elementary school and afternoons with regular students at the high school. "Sometimes he gets confused with his schedule but someone is always there to put him back on track." Once, when Pat has to be away, she asks that I pick him up after the one o'clock gym class. While waiting on the sidewalk for Pierre to come out, I am totally amazed at what I witness. Pierre is coming towards me seemingly unaware that he is surrounded by a little troop of bodyguards–two in the front, two at the back and one on each side. Apparently this is an ongoing practice with the students who take turns making sure he gets back to his class. It sure gives my heart a nice warm fuzzy feeling!

Reports from the various teachers in the year 1985 indicate that Pierre is adjusting to being off his medication. He seems less nervous and less irritable when having to deal with people. Unfortunately, his interest and attention span have not increased but he attempts to try. The teachers of the classes he attends during Pat's remedial work schedule state that he tries to participate, but not as well as he used to and that sometimes he falls asleep in class.

In 1986 and 1987 Pierre participates in all activities that Pat introduces, but his little heart does not seem to be part of it. Sometimes he rides his bike. We go together. How I wish I could make life better for him.

Thanks for your patience, Pat. You are awesome.

Pierre's Perspective

I call my new teacher P-Pat. I learn different things with her. But I'm not as I should be. I'm not like before. I'm not really part of the class.
My mind is not where I am. I can't concentrate. I'm up half the night–I can't sleep–I get up and put all the lights on.
It should be daytime and everybody should get up.
I forget to eat–Mamaman and Jin feed me. I laugh a lot.
I don't know what's wrong with me! I am in my own little world.
I am loved. I will survive.

VII

Age 19-33 1987–2001

Industrie Prairie Industries (IPI) Gravelbourg Workshop & Group Home

Mother's Perspective

We know that Pierre has to do something else after he leaves school. He also has to leave home eventually–it is a 'normal' way of life. Early in 1984 an enterprising group of Gravelbourg citizens, service clubs, community groups, and businesses, start working to set up a sheltered workshop for the disabled. Gilles is very much part of that group. On June 24, 1984, the Gravelbourg Bon Ami, Inc. Board is incorporated as a non-profit organization providing services to people with disabilities.

A needs survey of Gravelbourg and area (from Herbert/Chaplin to Crestwynd in the north, down to the U.S. border in the South, Mankota/Kincaid to the west and Assiniboia/Coronach to the east) is completed. The results serve as a basis for a proposal to the Government of Saskatchewan showing that funding for a sheltered workshop and group home for six people is warranted. Many meetings are held with the aforementioned organizations as government funding is conditional on a percentage of the cost being raised locally.

It is important to visit various workshops throughout the province to get ideas so the new board sets off for a one-week learning quest. To make conversation, Gilles, at one workshop, stops at the table of one of the clients and asks, "What do you do here?" She replies, as she demonstrates, that she is making flowers for weddings. Gilles picks one up, holds it to his nose and says, "Umm . . . does it ever smell good!" She pulls at his arm to get him closer and whispers, "It's plastic."

In March 1986, the Telemiracle Foundation of Saskatchewan gives Bon Ami, Inc. a substantial grant. The Ministry of Social Services in April approves a donation for the construction of the Sheltered Workshop and a Group Home to accommodate six people. A building on the outskirts of Gravelbourg, ideal in location and space, is purchased in October for a workshop by Bon Ami, Inc.

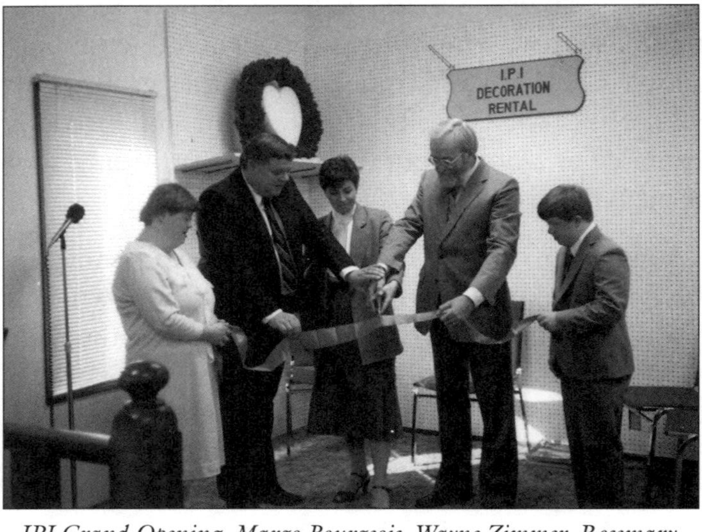

IPI Grand Opening. Margo Bourgeois, Wayne Zimmer, Rosemary Richmond, Manager, IPI, Ray Mulaire (Chair of Bon Ami, Inc.), and Pierre Piché

Everything is moving swiftly, thanks to the efficiency of the Board of Bon Ami, Inc. which is comprised of interested individuals and a representative from each organization.

April 1, 1987, Industrie Prairie Industries (IPI), the workshop component of Bon Ami, Inc. is in operation. On September 1, the first nine clients set foot in their new work and activity areas. At age 19, Pierre is one of these lucky people. I am so hoping this total change in his life will turn things around for him.

In September, seeing as there is a bit of highway to navigate, and the weather is beautiful, Pierre and I bike to the workshop. The Transit bus picks him up during the winter. Pierre seems happier. He's busy in the Activity Centre with rug hooking, macramé hangers, and flower-making for graduations and weddings. Staff find him very rigid in his routine and activities. They are amused as he refuses to allow time for coffee breaks!

The Grand Opening of IPI is scheduled for October 3, 1987. Our manager, Rosemary Richmond, asks me to coordinate the evening activities. I have always wanted to lip-sync to Dolly Parton's 'Nine-to-Five'–what a perfect opportunity!–not to mention that it is an excellent way to get the audience 'in the spirit of things'. *Le Mat du Collège Mathieu*, *l'Octopus*, ballerinas, tap and jazz dancers, and brilliant sax renditions by a native son all delight the audience. My sister, Alice, decides to lip-sync to Diane Dufresne and my other sister, JoAnne and our daughter, Valérie, both accomplished dancers, end the show with a bang. A totally successful grand opening! After the show, a client comes up to me and says, "Mrs. Piché, if you want to be Dolly Parton you will have to get bigger boobs." Shucks!!! and I thought I had endowed myself quite liberally!!!

Val brings our future son-in-law to the celebration. Thank goodness the above antics do not deter him from marrying Val in October 1988. The picture of Pierre in his tux on the back cover of this book was taken at this time.

On July 31, 1989, a sod-turning ceremony takes place to mark the beginning of construction for a group home. All the time the house is being built, we pop in occasionally and show Pierre where his room is going to be. “Look, Pierre, you’ll have a nice back yard view. Look at how big your closet is going to be. Do you think the bed should go here? And the dresser here?” I keep asking him. His little eyes speak volumes, showing interest, but, of course, no vocal answers are forthcoming.

The first clients move to the group home in January 1990. Pierre moves in February. He is 22 years old. The week before he moves, the manager, Rosemary, the staff, and I have a meeting at the house. All is going fine until it is mentioned that Pierre should not have contact with the family for about a month just to make sure he adapts. The tears start flowing. Staff join me.

When the time arrives for the move, he helps pack his belongings. I carry pants and shirts on hangers. We arrive at the house, hang up his clothes, and he refuses to come back home. I don’t have the courage to go back when Gilles and Rod move his dresser and bed. The same feelings of my threatened separation from Pierre as a baby are all back. A four-day migraine sets in and I have to talk to myself ‘big time’ that this *is* ‘best’ for him. He needs to be as independent in life as his brothers and sister. The ‘month’ ruling lasts two weeks. When we pick him up, he’s shy with us but finally warms up and gives a big smile.

Daniel gets married to Mary in July of 1990 and he asks his two brothers to be best men. Mary's friend, Liz, as Pierre's escort, is wonderful with him. No cushions to carry this time!

Does Pierre ever fall in love? Yes, he does. His first love is 'P-Pat'. The second is a lovely girl with Down's named Lana who sings continually and obviously works her way into my son's heart. Proof is as follows: IPI is going camping; I drop in at the workshop to wish Pierre a good trip; I see him with an arm around Lana's neck and I can tell he has eyes only for her. What a fantastic feeling to see him so happy. Eventually Lana and her family move away, but in the wings there is a staff member at IPI named Debbie. Whenever he hears Debbie's name his eyes just twinkle. Oh yes, I can safely say that my boy has been touched by the Lovebug.

Life at the group home is good for Pierre. We pick him up every Sunday for church and he spends the day with us. The odd time he takes a while to get out of the car when we return him to his house, but while that can be a little heart wrenching, basically, it is good. His eating habits actually improve, i.e., raw vegetables and various meats. The only way I can get him to eat these things is to put them in soup.

Pierre becomes an uncle in October of 1990. He is not impressed with Kristyn, a daughter for Val and Jim, when she visits Gravelbourg at Christmas. That this two-month-old treasure is passed around to the grandmas, myself, Gilles, is half bad, but when Rod picks her up, tears start streaming down his face. He has never had to share Rod before! But when Val and Jim return at Easter, all of a sudden Pierre takes Kristyn away from my mother and takes her to Rod. Obviously he is mending fences with his feelings. In 1992

Pierre becomes an uncle twice again–Monica, another daughter for Jim and Val, and Brandon, a son for Dan and Mary. There are no incidents this time.

I learn a new word–stimming–Pierre is doing repetitive actions with fingers and shoulders. A new stage in his life for us to contend with. Now that I look back, however, I realize that what he was doing as a baby–extending his arm as far as it would go–slowly moving it right to left–and watching his fingers on the arm's return trip was probably stimming, as well as the tongue sucking, playing with his hair and chewing on his thumb. So, I guess this is not new; there is just more of it!

Gilles, Pierre, and I meet regularly with IPI staff (workshop and group home) where ideas and comments are exchanged: Pierre's communication skills improve yearly; he is showing more independence in developing and dealing with interpersonal relationships; he participates in housekeeping duties and grocery shopping (even initiates these); makes coffee for staff and clients at the workshop; crushes cans for SARCAN (his favourite job), and attends various summer camps.

In 1990, there are incidents of Pierre kicking and slapping other clients. Intensive monitoring and talking to Pierre by all of us seems to put a stop to this behaviour.

Pierre has always been susceptible to colds and pneumonia in the months of November to February, so he is closely monitored during these months. In 1994, at age 26, his cholesterol levels are high. He is also overweight. A special diet including salmon, low carbohydrates, low fat–and no more chips and Coke–is enforced. Staff tell me that at one point they watch him inch his way to the cupboard keeping an eye on staff and quickly grab a cookie when he thinks they are not looking. "We didn't have the heart to take it away from him," they tell me. The worst offenders to the new rule is his two grandmothers, ***Mère*** and ***Pom***. The threat of not being allowed to see Pierre again

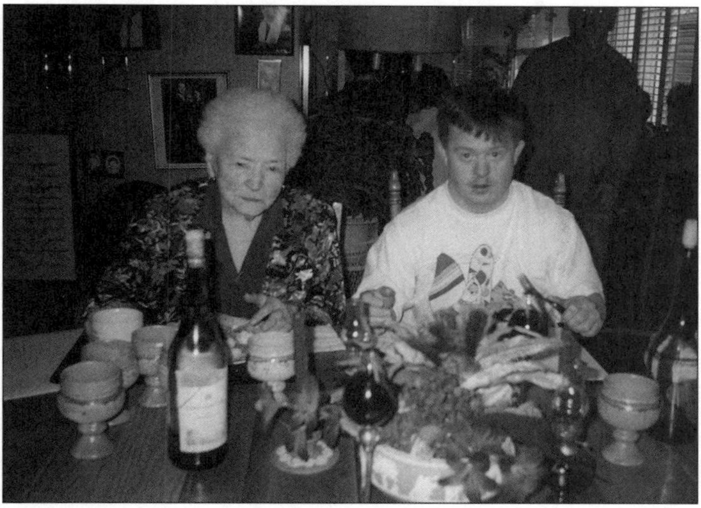

Pom and Pierre

finally gets the message across to the two culprits. They also know that Pierre tattles when he gets chips and/or Coke!

After the deaths of his grandfathers, the ritual is for the two grandmas to come for breakfast on Sundays; then Pierre walks them back home. What a picture! Each grandmother on either side of Pierre walking arm-in-arm–Pierre at 4'11", my mother not much taller and my mother-in-law just over five feet. My mother is in her 70s and my mother-in-law in her 80s.

During this time, too, we start noticing that Pierre is slowing down. Every Sunday for years it has been his responsibility to clear the table after breakfast. Now we notice that activity takes him a lot longer to complete. He doesn't seem to respond as readily to what is going on around him. Is the dieting causing him to change? Adjustments are also made at the group home to accommodate this slower pace, i.e., allowing more time for bathing, eating, etc.

My mother does not start 1997 very well. Her heart is giving her problems. After a stint in the hospital, we move her to the Gravelbourg Foyer d'Youville where she gets the ultimate of care. Pierre often visits and, of course, gives her a big kiss. He's now sporting a moustache and mom says, "Pierre, that tickles." So he gives her another one. Obviously he feels it's an invitation.

During my daily visits with Mom at the Foyer I bring her up to date on how I'm progressing in the baking/house cleaning departments in preparation for Rod and Isabelle's wedding on July 12. I am totally ready.

Mom dies on July 4, 1997, at the age of 80. She had specified her wishes for her funeral, one being that she is to be cremated and Pierre is to carry her in and out of church. I explain to Pierre, "***Mère*** is gone to see ***Jésus*** and it's OK." Pierre carries her in and out of church and sits the urn on his knees as we travel to the cemetery. After the funeral, guests gather at our house. Pierre sits beside ***Pom*** and holds her hand for a very long time.

Mére is pretty sneaky. I'm sure she planned her departure from this world so that close family members who had answered they couldn't come to the wedding are now all in attendance. It is time for rejoicing and dancing as we welcome Isabelle to the family.

Gilles and I start traveling, staying away for up to seven weeks at a time, so Pierre is more on his own. Rod, being the closest in distance often pops in for visits. According to staff, Pierre seems to handle our absences well.

In October 1997 Pierre is started on Eltroxin due to an inactive thyroid. In time, we all see a shift again, for the better. Pierre is more aware, he moves a little faster–a participant in life again. His weight, between 110 and 115, is maintained. In springtime, he rides his bike or walks to the workshop from the group home which is not far. I wish I would have known sooner that his thyroid was a problem!

Nine months after my mother, Grandmother Piché, *(Pom)* passes away in May 1998. This time Pierre does not hold hands with anyone. Both his precious grandmothers are now gone. It's hard to know what he is feeling.

Physical aggression returns with a vengeance at various periods. He initiates confrontations by slapping or kicking. He does not discriminate–you get a hit even if he loves you. Staff members are not immune to it. I, too, am the recipient of a couple of his slaps. To be fair, he has also been at the

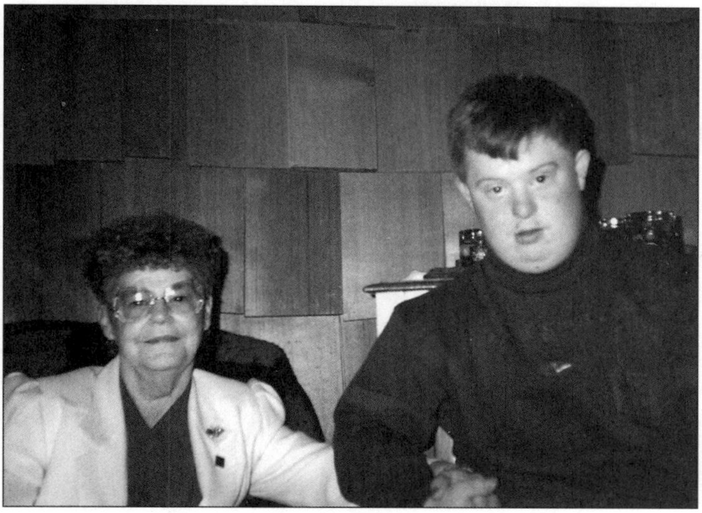

Mére and Pierre

receiving end of such treatment from another client, which does not excuse his actions. Written reports of every act of aggression is shared between ourselves as parents and staff at the workshop and group home. Gilles and I decide to bring Pierre home every Friday night and bring him back to the workshop on Monday mornings. This seems to help reduce some of his frustration.

I make contact through the Internet to various organizations that are knowledgeable about Down syndrome behaviour; so does Rosemary, the manager of IPI. The Internet provided a lot of information but I still didn't feel that I was getting answers; maybe it's because I didn't know what questions to ask!

Gilles, Pierre and I travel to Saskatoon in February 2001, to meet with a member of the Department of Psychiatry. No resolution is arrived at.

One revealing piece of advice I receive is from a Grey Nun sister. She worked many years with the disabled in St. Amant Centre in Winnipeg and is now stationed in Gravelbourg. When I bring up Pierre's behaviour she says, "Oh, Pierre is not happy where he is. He is ready for a change." I ask her to pray for some kind of solution. What is our alternative?

Pierre's Perspective

(As I am not constantly with Pierre any more I find it more difficult to read his thoughts, his feelings.)

VIII

Age 33 2001

Medicine Hat, Alberta

Mother's Perspective

Every now and then throughout our 39 years of marriage, Gilles and I get on a kick of 'let's build a new house', and we put our house on the market. We usually end up taking the For Sale sign off because I love my house and I change my mind. But 2001 is different. We actually purchase a lot in the newest crescent in Gravelbourg; my 'dream' plans are sitting on the dining room table, and my mind works overtime placing appliances, furniture and book shelves.

A date to remember–April 17, 2001: it's Easter weekend and Pierre is recovering from a very bad bout of pneumonia–his third since his birth. Val, Jim and the girls from Calgary, and Rod and Isabelle from Swift Current, have just arrived in time to attend the Good Friday services. As we sit around waiting to leave for the 3:00 services, the phone rings. It's the real estate agent. "If you're still interested in selling, I have a buyer."

Mixed emotions–happiness, a feeling of loss, a sense of adventure, seem to run through all of us. Needless to say, all our memories have been lived in this house–family gatherings, baptisms, first communions, confirmations, graduations, weddings, funerals, Christmases. We call Dan and Mary in Sudbury. Long distance sharing is important. We sell.

Pierre recuperates nicely from his pneumonia and is back at work and in the group home. His life is stable; ours is hectic.

By the end of April we move into a two-bedroom apartment. The apartment is cute but confining. On May 3, Gilles and I decide to take a little trip to Calgary with a stop over at Terry and Aimé's who have recently moved to Medicine Hat.

Being me, I like to be in total control of my life and what happens around me. The month of May teaches me a lesson.

On arrival in Medicine Hat we visit a cousin and get a WOW experience when we see their condo — we check with the real estate agent to see show homes to get ideas for our new home — have to confess to agent after visiting condos that we are not really interested — when he asks, "And why not?" we answer — " because we have a handicapped son and we don't go any where without him"— agent makes inquiries — agent hands me the phone — I like the sound of this person's voice — we meet her at 9:00 the next morning — I not only like her voice, but we like her message which lasts over an hour — the name of the Association is CORE — there would be a place for Pierre at the workshop and in a residence — she mentions other workshops/organizations available in Medicine Hat — there seems to be a lot happening in this city for the mentally challenged — she mentions Special Olympics — Pierre is a good swimmer — "would he be interested in joining?" — we leave CORE — I feel "whatever" to the depth of my bones — we don't go to Calgary — we go back to Gravelbourg.

It is seeding time anyway. Gilles and I bring up what is available for Pierre in Medicine Hat. Maybe he needs a major change. Remember what Sister said about Pierre not being happy?

Ten days later we are back in Medicine Hat–this time with Rod. We need another opinion. We meet the same young lady from CORE. Rod says, "Yes, this would be good for Pierre" — go back to the real estate agent — all houses that we had looked at are sold — well, maybe except for one which is in 'pending until their house is sold' mode — we put a deposit on it — May 28, it is ours — July 29, 2001, we are Medicine Hatters; we are Albertans!

At the beginning of June I recognize that I'm not in control, I decide to let go and just enjoy the ride. We definitely are meant to be here.

All through July and August, Pierre is with us. All we hear is, "Francis . . ."–an ex-roommate at the Gravelbourg Group Home–to the point where Isabelle teasingly says, "Pierre, I don't want to hear the "F" word any more." I haven't figured out if Francis means the actual person or the workshop and group home. But obviously he misses where he was. I keep him busy helping me place things in the new house.

Arrangements for Pierre to be at CORE (i.e. acceptance, funding, space) are achieved precisely and efficiently. Pierre starts work on September 1. Gilles and I take turns driving him to and from work. He seems happy to pack his lunch and there are smiles when we drop him off. We meet the staff person who will be in charge of the residence–her name is Pam. The interaction between them seems to be good. I like her.

It is the first of October and time for Pierre to move into the residence.

What is my problem? Those same feelings of 'letting him go' are back again. Do these feelings exist because of the threatened separation after his birth, or is it because he is mentally deficient? I can't figure it out! But they are real.

Gilles and I watch Pierre practise for the Special Olympics swim team. We watch him bowl. His Monday evenings are spent at the Friendship Centre. Staff tell me that the first Monday he is there, he approaches the microphone after being introduced. No one understands what he is saying. Is he speaking French? However, he insists that speaking or singing in the mike is part of the weekly routine. I love it.

Because Pierre has never been taught the strokes of swimming, it becomes obvious that he needs one-on-one training. Pam takes up the challenge. To date, out of the five events that he has competed in against Lethbridge, Red Deer, Airdrie, Calgary, Brooks, sometimes Edmonton, he has brought home firsts, seconds or thirds quite a few times. Good job, Pam. Pierre is so enjoying this.

Gilles and I reiterate how good this move is in many ways. Pierre likes his roommates, Jason and Paul. They seem to like him. Gilles and I like the families of Paul and Jason, and that's very important to us. Through CORE, Pierre volunteers in the community i.e. at senior citizen homes,

Food Bank, delivering mail, etc. Staff also try to teach him street safety. He attends sessions at the YMCA regularly for exercises. Pierre appears happy, both at work and at the residence.

For Gilles and I it is important that after our deaths, Pierre never becomes a burden to his siblings. This move to Medicine Hat situates Pierre right in the middle of Rodrigue, two hours away in Swift Current, and Valérie, two hours and forty minutes away in Calgary. From this distance they can monitor Pierre's existence and not have him hamper their lives and that of their families.

After the first two weeks of October Pierre seems to be happily established and it is time for Gilles and I to enjoy our new home and surroundings.

So why am I feeling 'unsettled' again, or incomplete, or not . . . whatever?!! Maybe it's because everything is new!

By mid November Gilles is growing lumps–neck, groin, behind the ear–that one is painful. The doctor orders tests — November 22 Gilles is diagnosed with Hodgkins Lymphoma — early December we have an appointment at the Tom Baker Centre in Calgary — cancer is found in the bone marrow as well — it is now called Non-Hodgkins Lymphoma — the first treatment is given that day; five more are to be given in Medicine Hat a month apart depending on how the little white cells are behaving. April 25, 2002, Gilles passes away at 3:25 p.m.

When Pierre walks in to the Medicine Hat Hospital, I explain, "Gilles is gone to see *Jésus*, and it's OK." He sits by Gilles and holds his hand. Every now and then he gets up and gives him a big kiss; then sits again and holds his hand.

Even though we have moved, our plans are that we be cremated and buried in Gravelbourg. On May 4, 2002, I honour Gilles' wish. Pierre and I travel to Swift Current and then to Gravelbourg with Gilles' urn between us. I talk about Gilles, and Pierre looks at me and listens.

I ask Piché-Hawkins Funeral Home to reserve front row seats at the Cathedral for the 15 people coming from Medicine Hat, including Jason and Paul, as well as for those attending from IPI. It is a beautiful ceremony with much family participation. Pierre is Urn Bearer. During the mass, Pierre gets up and goes to get Pam so she can sit beside us. I read that as meaning, "Pam, you are part of my family." And to me, that is very, very good.

Since our move to Medicine Hat the ritual is to pick Pierre up at his residence Sunday morning so he can spend the day with us. On the first Sunday that Pierre and I are by ourselves, we come back from church and Pierre sets the table for three. When I break down, Pierre comes up quickly and gives me a humongous hug. Good timing, Big Guy!

For a time, whenever we are in the car together, he says, *"Jin"*–probably remembering our trip with the Urn. So I ask him, "*Où Gilles?* –Where is Gilles?" He answers, *"Avec, Jésus* – With Jesus*"*. Then I say, "Right. Now it's Pierre and Maman, and it's OK." He smiles.

When we go to Gravelbourg from Medicine Hat, we pass the cemetery as it is right beside the highway. Pierre always points and says *"Jin"*. I say, "Yes, let's have a visit with Gilles." We both touch the columbarium.

In August 2002, Pam moves to England–a job transfer for her husband. I worry that Pierre will have a reaction. So far, so good.

Pierre has lost many favourite people in his 34 years. He seems to adjust to each loss. However, if I should go as quickly as Gilles, I must assure myself that he is secure in his residence which is peopled with excellent staff and great 'roomies'. Through the variety at CORE and its community involvement, I know his interest in life will be maintained and closely monitored by staff. Since Gilles has died, Pierre calls me every day when he returns from work. Of course I talk and he answers "uh, uh." Then I say, "Kiss." He answers with a big smack. I say, "Love you," and most of the time he clearly replies, "Love you." I thank God every day for his presence in my life.

Pierre's Perspective

I am loved. I know it. I am happy.

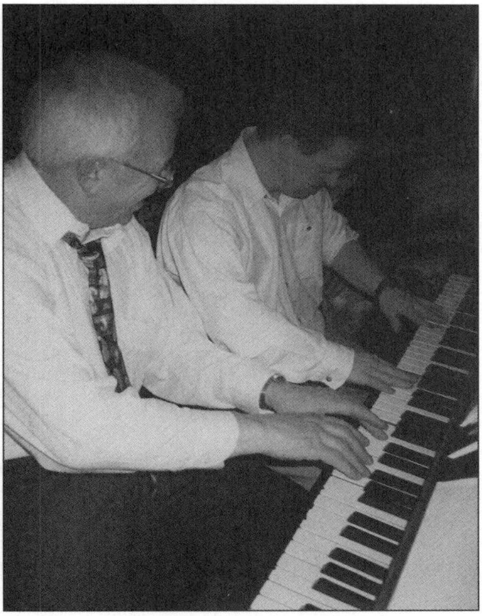

Pierre and Gilles perform (neither knows how to play)

Epilogue

Gilles and I married in 1962. He had no objections to having six children. At the time he was working for Manulife and was traveling quite a bit for the company all through southern Saskatchewan. By the time the fourth pregnancy happened, his dad decided to retire and Gilles took over as grain elevator agent. He felt it was time to stay home and help raise the kids. My contribution to the working world before marriage was as a legal secretary, in Gravelbourg, in Montreal, and then back to Gravelbourg again. I loved my work.

The six children never happened because we did not know how difficult it would be to raise a handicapped child. Pierre is a total joy in our lives, as are our three other children. I sometimes wonder why Pierre went into his crisis, his depression. Is there anything we could have done differently? Most people with Down syndrome do not seem to suffer that fate. I'm happy for that.

He is OK again and I really feel that our move to Medicine Hat is a 'plus' in his life. He loves to swim, which he does two to three times a week–with Special Olympics and with staff at the residence; skates during the winter months; attends hockey games and takes long walks in the many parks. His contentment here in Medicine Hat does not take anything away from IPI in Gravelbourg–which is a well run organization with great staff and interesting clients. At IPI Pierre learned how to be more independent from us. It's just that Sister was probably correct. Pierre needed a change, a new challenge.

I am not aware if the two other children whose birth was questionable when Pierre was born were Down syndrome or not.

I know that Doc probably explained about the extra chromosome that becomes part of the makeup of a Down syndrome at conception. However, at the time of his initial visit I don't remember. I read a lot about the syndrome after Pierre's birth when I was trying to figure out why this happens.

I have answered the 'why me?' feeling I had for so many months after Pierre was born in this way: Pierre was given to us for a purpose. Gilles never questioned 'why me?', but I suppose being who, what I am, I need to search why things happen in my life. The reason I have come up with is that none of us knew what having a child with challenges was all about . . . family, friends, maybe even the community. It was up to me, to us, to bring that to light and make the presence of these special people known and validated. I also feel that many people's lives are different because of Pierre . . . and all for the better.

Did our marriage suffer? In the 'dark days' before we got on the same page and started working together, it was a bit tough. Then again, which marriage doesn't suffer a major storm only to enjoy smoother waters thereafter?

Did Daniel, Valérie, Rodrigue suffer because of Pierre? I think they are compassionate, well-adjusted, loving individuals who have good relationships with their spouses and children. What more can one ask?

Pierre has always been well accepted by his cousins on both sides of the family. Chloé, Guylaine's daughter, is fascinated by Pierre. When she started walking, she would go to him and extend her arms, waiting for him to pick her up. She wouldn't move until he paid attention. We had to say, "Pierre, Chloé needs a hug". He would pick her up, give the hug and quickly put her down. Now, in 2003, she is three and she hops on his lap and looks at him. He's not sure what to do so he smiles at her. One time, we were at a hockey game in Gravelbourg and IPI clients were all there supporting their favourite team. Chloé noticed another person with Down's and she said, "Pierre, look, there's another you." I am always amazed how very young children pick up there is something different about Pierre.

As it wasn't 'my turn' to have the family celebrations for Christmas, 2002, Pierre and I flew to Sudbury, Ontario. Pierre met a new little nephew, Josh, for the first time–another son for Dan and Mary. Pierre occasionally paid attention to him. Rod and Isabelle are expecting their first child in 2004. It will be interesting to see Pierre's reaction.

Information coming out on Down syndrome behaviour indicates that they age more quickly than we 'normal' people do. This can range from between 20 and 30 years. I always tease Pierre that we are about the same age. Other information indicates that it is also very likely he will develop Alzheimer's.

No matter. I live in the present and I am always open to learn what Pierre has to teach me . . . patience and 'slow down, Mom' are two major ones. I know I'll be practising for a long time! No problem!

It is unfortunate that I completed this book after Gilles is gone. I know he would have loved to share his point of view.

When we moved to Medicine Hat, Gilles was elected to the CORE board in September 2001. In Gravelbourg, we used to take turns being on the IPI board–it is important that parents be part of the decision-making. I felt that eventually I would take my turn when he completed his term at CORE. At the Annual General Meeting in September 2002, I was elected to the board of CORE–it was already my turn.

TESTIMONIALS

MY OLD CHAP

Daniel, *Brother*

There once was a billionaire from Texas who wanted to make sure that people visited his grave site. Before he died he had a bank machine installed at his future grave site. When the billionaire died, he had already given all his closest friends a bank card. Whenever his friends would come to visit his grave, they would swipe the card in the bank machine and a one hundred dollar bill would come out.

If Pierre Piché was to emulate the actions of this Texas billionaire, he would have installed a Coca-Cola machine instead of a bank machine. Pierre loves his Coke and he would want all his closest friends and relatives to savour the one drink that satisfies his taste buds to the fullest.

The symbolism behind Pierre's choice in Coca-Cola is astonishing. The Coca-Cola Company trades on the NYSE under the symbol KO. This company is one of the biggest companies in the world with annual sales that exceed twenty billion dollars. If you compare this company to my small business, there's no comparison. When you compare the soul of Pierre Piché to my soul, once again there's no comparison.

When Pierre Piché came to this earth on August 18, 1968, his soul was at the higher end of the continuum. My research has taught me that all mentally and physically

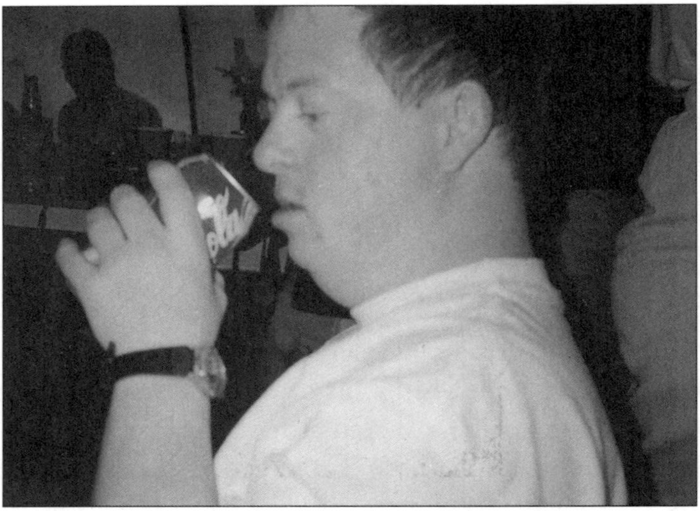

"The pause that refreshes"

challenged individuals that enter this physical world have spirits that are more evolved than the spirit of the average person like myself.

To this day, every once in a while when I'm sitting alone in my backyard having a cold Coca-Cola, I raise my glass to the sky and I say. "This is for you old chap."

MY TEDDY BEAR, MY FRIEND

Valérie, *Sister*

Pierre is my youngest brother and is special because he is Down syndrome. People knew he was different because of his looks and he attended a special class at school.

Pierre is a good listener. I can tell him all kinds of things and he never gets tired of listening to me. He is like a big teddy bear, always my friend, and always there to give me a hug when I need one.

Pierre has taught me how to teach. Being three years older, I remember sitting with him and trying to help him read. How exciting when he remembered the word. I was determined to keep going so he would be the best reader that he could be.

Mom and Dad were always open about Pierre. I guess I can say that is why it has always made me so proud to share what Pierre is all about. I find people very interesting. When Pierre and I go out I notice how many stares he gets. I feel like reaching out to everyone so I can tell them all about Pierre and assure them not to be scared.

Pierre was someone I wanted to take care of. He and I usually went to visit my Grandma and Grandpa after school. They were always happy to see us both. Their love for Pierre made me love him even more. When we'd leave they'd say, "We'll see you tomorrow." Mom and Dad often went out on weekends therefore my brothers and I took care of Pierre. Rod and I usually had arguments on where Pierre would sleep. We both wanted Pierre all to ourselves.

Photography

When Mom gave me her camera I fell in love with photography. Pierre loved getting his picture taken and I loved snapping pictures. Pierre and I would take turns taking pictures. We're still doing this.

Swimming

One of Pierre's talents is swimming. I could never figure out how he could hold his breath from one end of the pool to the other. When friends commented on this, I'd always tell them how much he likes the water and how comfortable he is in it.

Patience

Pierre has taught us patience. I'd like to share this episode of when we were younger. It is Sunday morning and we're all getting ready for church. Pierre is not a fast mover. It seems when you try to rush him he gets slower. This particular Sunday we got up late and Pierre hadn't had his chocolate milk and toast yet. Pierre has to eat every last crumb and drink to the very last drop. Oh, my gosh!! It's pretty funny now. Dad is in the car waiting as patiently as he can–backing up the car–commenting, "How come Mom didn't get Pierre ready in time?" Dan and I are in the car; finally Pierre and Mom get in. Dad says, "Well, where's Rod?" Sometimes I think Pierre taught Rod how to move slowly. If I remember correctly, after a few Sunday mornings like this, Pierre wasn't allowed to have a full breakfast before church. And Rod probably had to move quicker, too!

Friends

My friends often asked me, "Does Pierre understand what you are saying?" Some would comment: "Isn't it too bad that he's handicapped?" "You probably wish you would have had a sister." This came up quite often when I was growing up and it always kind of hurt me. How could they say that when they didn't know what Pierre was all about? That kind of comment always made my love for Pierre stronger. I always thought that maybe if they had been raised with a handicap child they would have understood better what these people are all about.

Now, as an adult, married with two children, I imagine it may have been really hard for my parents, as a couple, to raise three young children and a baby with Down's–not knowing what that affliction was all about. I commend them on all their hard work, their devotion, to make Pierre the best person that he can be. They have showed me how to love and be proud of my brother, Pierre. I am not the only one that has benefited from this, but all family, friends and strangers who were interested in knowing about him. I realize that people who weren't brought up with a challenged child in the family look at the handicapped in a totally different way.

I hope I can pass on the understanding of Down syndrome to other people as my parents have. I know my husband and children look at Pierre and people like him in a positive way, probably because I am so open about Pierre.

MY FRIEND, MY WRESTLING BUDDY

Rodrigue, ***Brother***

As families evolve, you hear about the bonding that takes place among siblings. This family is no exception. Many great memories over the years have been shared. No doubt the closeness that Pierre and I developed over the years is because we were only two years apart. After the other two left Gravelbourg to pursue their studies, Pierre and I had more time together.

Growing up, I never considered Pierre different from anybody else. He was someone I could talk to–he's a great listener, was someone I could wrestle with, and still do, was and is still very strong. Down syndrome, yes, but did his lack of abilities change the way I perceived him when he was around me, my family, my friends? No, to me he was simply Pierre, my brother, nothing more, nothing less. Mom and Dad always said, "Make sure you stick up for Pierre, just like Valérie and Daniel did for you." That I did. I consider him a close friend who at times needs my help and protection.

Childhood memories are plentiful: bike riding and skateboarding (we made many miles–our cousin, Paul, Pierre and I), Special Olympics in Gravelbourg, vocabulary cards, Pierre's graduation picture, playing street hockey, etc.

One episode comes to mind. In our pre-teenage days, rock picking on the farm was a Saturday ritual. We would all leave with Dad early in the morning, all cuddled up in the front seat of the half-ton truck, and not come back to town until late afternoon. Mornings flew by. We filled and unloaded the back of the truck many times. Lunchtime rolled around. Mom had prepared sandwiches, snacks, and sent a couple of water jugs. All of us kids were assigned a job. Val was the truck driver, Dan and Rod were the rock pickers. Dad, the scout, seemed to spot the stones from a mile away. Pierre, who accompanied Val in the front seat, had it all figured out. Sure, he picked stones when hilltops were plentiful, but it appeared to be his job to make sure he had *his* share of the water. Never did we make it back to town having a drop left in any of the water coolers! To this day, a couple of water jugs is nearly never enough.

Harvest time is always such fun and it gives me great satisfaction to call Pierre and ask him to join me in the fall work. He never refuses.

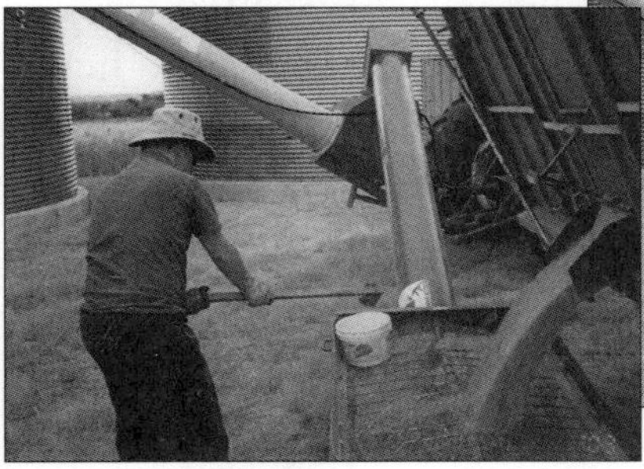

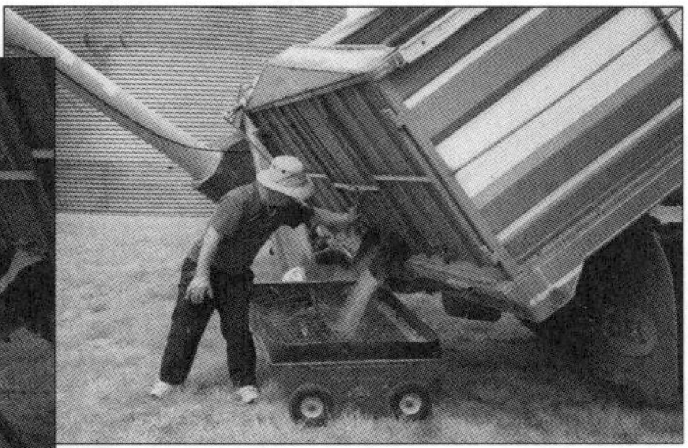

"Doing what I've been trained to do"

One great thing about Pierre is when you show him how to do a task you know he will always do it the same way. I taught him how to sample grain from the truck. With many years of grain sampling experience under his belt, I sense this is the reason why he accompanies me for harvest. He enjoys sitting next to me in the grain truck. His right arm sits on the passenger door and extends to the outside. He is smiling ear to ear. He's dressed in farm clothes, wearing his work gloves, and waits for the grain truck to be loaded from the combine so he can do the job I trained him for when we get to the bins.

As an added bonus, he loves the time of day when lunch arrives so he can eat in the field and drink his Coke. To add to his fun filled day, nothing can top hearing him ask to go to the bathroom, like men can do on the farm, in the open air. After the duty is performed he quickly returns to his post. A big grin on his face.

I often wonder what my life would be without Pierre. I know I probably would not have experienced the true meaning of patience, or the joy of giving and sharing.

As the years unfold, with Pierre establishing himself in Medicine Hat, another chapter is evolving. Just in the short time he has moved to Alberta, I have witnessed a new side of him that I am certainly proud of, and certainly have never experienced before: his independence and the decisions he makes with confidence. For example, on one of my impromptu visits at his workshop, at CORE, on an early Friday afternoon, just after lunch, he is sitting, his back to me, colouring. I walk up behind him, he has not noticed me yet. I start talking to his neighbour, and all of a sudden, as he hears my voice, he stands up, turns around, and gives me a big hug. I chat with him. After a few minutes, he leads me by the hand to show me his swimming bag next to his locker. His way of saying, "I will be going swimming after work." He is very excited. Then he pulls out his lunch bag from his locker, then pulls out a banana. I insist he put it back in the bag and locker since I am sure he has just eaten lunch. As I continue to chat with him, he leads me by the hand to another room. I'm not sure if I should be letting him, not knowing if staff permits this, but I am impressed with his authority to lead, so I let him. We end up in the painting room where he wants to show me water paintings he has spent time on. Staff reaches on a shelf and hands a binder of all the students' pictures. Pierre, after seating himself, smiling, opens the binder and insists I view them with him. I am fascinated. Soon after, someone in the hallway yells, 'coffee time'; it did not take Pierre one second before he hops off his chair and grabs my hand. He takes me over to his locker, grabs the banana from his lunch bag, always holding my hand and walks to the cafeteria. He lets my hand go, places the banana on an open table, walks to the beverage counter and pours himself a glass of water; comes back to the table, places the glass next to his banana, and turns to me. I am not sure what he will do next. He gives me a hug and sits down. I took that to mean: "Thanks for coming, it was nice seeing you; sorry, it's my coffee break!" I love to see this streak of independence in him and the authority that comes with it.

When I heard Pierre was involved in Special Olympic swimming, I promised myself that I would try and commit to most of his meets. Thinking back from the early Special Olympic years, back in the 1970s, wow, what a thrill to be part of something like that again.

Would I change anything? No. I would not have wanted it to be any different. My life has been an eventful experience and I feel blessed to have Pierre share it with me. To sum it all up, Pierre has taught me to celebrate the little things in life.

My buddy, you have a fan for life!

Mary, *Sister-in-law*

Living 2000 miles away makes it difficult to really get to know Pierre. The first time I met him was at Valérie's wedding in 1988. He couldn't talk much but it seemed like people that were close to him understood him well. It's very noticeable that he likes chips and Coke, and likes to hold the remote control when we are watching TV. I try to score points by giving it to him whenever someone else has it. It works a little.

A visit from Gilles and Henriette accompanied by Pierre once or twice a year to Northern Ontario offers me a glimpse of who he is. Sometimes this is accompanied by a feeling of failure because, for whatever reason, I don't know how to get through.

In December 2002, Pierre and Henriette visited for Christmas. Gilles is no longer with us. Out of the blue Pierre gets up, walks across the room and gives me a big hug and kiss. I feel he finally knows who I am. It is a wonderful feeling.

Kristyn Bell, *Pierre's niece (12 years old when written)*

My uncle is handicapped. His name is Pierre Piché. He is very special to me. He isn't just an uncle; he's like a friend, a brother. Pierre has taught me over the years not to be afraid of mentally handicapped people. In my perspective, I find handicap people kind, great friends who listen to all your problems and are always there for you. When I was born 12 years ago on October 17, 1990, Pierre was there holding me very carefully. He can't pronounce my name so he calls me 'Kikin'. As I grow older I love Pierre even more and understand him. I hold his hand when we go places. He's my buddy. I love him very much. When I come to visit my grandma, Henriette Piché, he is usually there. Sometimes I get lucky and he has to go to one of his activities, like bowling, swimming and other great stuff he does. When I'm 20 years old I will remember Pierre as my uncle, my friend and a brother.

Monica, *Pierre's niece*
(7 years old when written)

Hi, my name is Monica Piché Bell. I am the daughter of Valérie Carmelle Piché.

I felt uncomfortable with Pierre because I didn't grow up with him but now I feel much more comfortable because I'm used to him.

At first I was really scared (very scared). I was scared because handicap people look different than us. And I couldn't understand what he was saying. When he came to hug me my gut felt scared and uncomfortable. If I had to introduce Pierre to my friends this is what I would say to make them comfortable: "This is my mother's brother which turns out to be my uncle. He is very nice so you don't have to worry."

What I like about Pierre is that he is a very, very good hugger.

Monique Piché,
Pierre's aunt

Pierre was born in 1968. At that time, I was living in the Arctic so I did not have the joy of seeing him often in early childhood, but I remember a particular summer holiday where Henriette, Pierre and I often went to Thompson Lake, eight miles south of Gravelbourg. Henriette creatively found ways of catching his attention to prompt him to speak. His joy was obvious as she sang his name *Pi-er-re* on different melodies, developing a bond between her and her special child.

One of the beautiful memories I have of Pierre is at Mom and Dad's 50th wedding anniversary in 1977. All the family members had been invited to do a skit or a song. Pierre, with the help of his mother, had practiced two songs: 'How much is that doggie in the window?' and *'Hier au soir sur mon perron, y'avait un beau ti minou'*. He had learned to say, 'Woof woof' or *'Miaou'* at the appropriate time. On the evening of the celebration, Pierre went on stage, held the mike and when his mother sang, 'How much is that doggie in the window?' he said, *'Miaou'*. He received a thunderous applause and bowed profusely. He had stolen the show! I remember Brigitte, Raymond's wife, saying, "Pierre is so authentic. He doesn't wear a mask."

Over the years, Pierre continued to become his own person and to develop his potential. In his early teens, he had a vocabulary of at least 50 words. He taught me one word that comes back to my mind on occasion. It's 'gildie' which means, 'Excuse me'.

He learned to be a ladies' man. He used to offer his arm to 'Pom' to help her cross the street. He loves to give gentle hugs and knows how to be a 'charmer'. His winning smile seems to say: "Isabelle, I'll win your heart like Rodrigue," "Mère, Pom, you will not be able to resist giving me a Coke," "Henriette, you're my favourite Mom," "Gilles, can I sit on your lap like I used to?"

He is an athlete. While very young, he learned to roll on a skateboard while sitting on it, to drive a two-wheel bike in town and a three-wheeler on the farm. He swims like a fish and he can stay underwater longer than you and I together. Since he moved to Medicine Hat he has learned new swimming techniques and goes bowling regularly. I've seen him enjoy looking at wrestling matches on TV and then try to do the same with Daniel and Rodrigue. He could have won a race at the Olympic Games once, but when he saw that the other racers were far behind, he stopped and waited for them to catch up to him!

At school, Pierre developed his artistic talents: he made cards, mosaics, rugs, flowers and drawings. Everyone knew and loved Pierre. He commanded respect. He allowed himself to be loved and even 'protected' by his friends. He used to beam whenever a friend came to get him to go to school. At home, he learned to share household tasks. As he grew older and went to 'live on his own' in a group home, he 'earned his living' by setting off to work each day, lunch pail in hand. Lately he has added volunteer work to his many activities.

Pierre could not have become who he is today without the love and commitment of his parents, Gilles and Henriette, his brothers and sister, Daniel, Valérie and Rodrigue, his extended family, his grandparents, especially Mère and Pom and his teachers and caregivers. Those closest to him were able to grasp his needs beyond words. They have done all they could so that Pierre could ‘bloom’ and be happy.

Pierre is a great gift to our family. He teaches us about ‘being’. He reminds us that what counts in life is not power, possessions or knowledge. He reminds us that the only true richness in life is loving relationships.

JoAnne (Shoshoi) Hartney,
Pierre's aunt

Pierre and I have an age difference of 13 years. From the day of his birth I enjoyed looking after him. He always makes me smile and laugh.

When I was in high school I had the opportunity to take a seminar in Saskatoon from specialists who taught rhythmics to groups of people who worked with children that were blind, mute or mentally challenged. The form of rhythmics they taught was to listen to the different beats of music and to keep rhythm by clapping hands, doing different steps with the feet, and eventually coordinating the routines together. I would then go with my friend, Barbara, once a week to Pierre's class to work with him and his classmates by doing routines that I had learnt or we had made up. The students seemed to enjoy themselves while doing the routines.

When I first brought John home (who is now my husband of 24 years) to meet the family, Pierre liked him instantly. He would connect the two of us together by saying both of our names together: *JoAnne-n-John*. Pierre seems to know who he feels comfortable with and who accepts him for the person he is.

Pierre was the ringbearer at our wedding and he was accompanied by his cousin, Guylaine, as flowergirl. Pierre was eleven years old and Guylaine was nine. Even with the age difference they were both the same height. Pierre was dressed in a black tuxedo and Guylaine in a white frilly dress. They were a cute couple. The day of the wedding Pierre did exactly as the job required, walking up the aisle carrying the heart pillow with the rings well attached. When it was time for group pictures to be taken Pierre was nowhere to be found. Some of the wedding party went out looking for him. They found him riding his bicycle around town wearing his tuxedo.

Having Pierre in my life made me confident to coach rhythmic gymnastics to the Special Olympians in Regina for six years. It was rewarding and a great opportunity for myself.

Thanks, Pierre.

Alain Piché, *Pierre's uncle*

Pierre's story needed to be told. Who could have done better than the one who bore him in her womb, nourished him and followed him every step of the way?

When Pierre was born on August 18, 1968, I was teaching at Collège Mathieu, an Oblate College in Gravelbourg. For the next eight years I would be stationed in Gravelbourg. As a brother and brother-in-law, I would have the privilege to often visit at Pierre's home and get to know Pierre. We were a closely knit family and Gilles and Henriette have always opened wide their welcoming arms.

Circumstances would have it that I was invited to lend a helping hand. I was very happy to do so as it brought me even closer to the family, helped me have a greater understanding of a challenged child, and an appreciation of the family dynamics that would evolve after Pierre's birth.

Henriette rightly puts the following words in Pierre's mouth: "I am loved, I will survive." To my mind, this saying could also be applied to all the members of Pierre's immediate family. Both parents were endowed with deep human and spiritual values and convictions which they then communicated to their children: compassion, openness, faith, courage, love, determination, service to the community and family bonds, to name but a few.

I was always deeply touched by the way Gilles and Henriette faced the challenge of accepting and journeying the best they could with a handicapped child, and at the same time keeping intact the bonds with the other siblings. It took a lot of courage, determination and creativity to open the mentality at the community, school, and governmental levels in order that the mentally handicapped would be recognized, accepted and given their rightful place. I, myself, have been the recipient through it all of a better understanding and acceptance that is helping me in my present ministry with the handicapped residents at the Taché Nursing Center in St. Boniface, Manitoba.

In the epilogue of her book, Henriette states: "Many people's lives are different because of Pierre." Indeed Pierre, in his own way, was the occasion of growth and development in his immediate family, his extended family, the school system, the town dynamics and the governmental agencies, all brought about by the energetic and insightful endeavours of his parents and other helpful hands. Yes, Pierre has been a blessing to all. At 35 years of age, he is a loving, compassionate, joyful and well-adjusted man who will continue to make his way into the hearts of those he meets. All that thanks to Gilles (who has now passed away) and especially to Henriette, Pierre's mother, who has courageously sustained Pierre every step of the way in his ups and downs.

PIERRE, MY GODSON

Alice Préfontaine, *Pierre's aunt*

I was so excited when my sister Henriette and Gilles asked if I would like to be godmother for their next child, number four. I couldn't wait for this baby to be born.

The big day came. Mom called to let me know that Henriette and Gilles had a baby boy. His name was to be Pierre. She also mentioned that there was something wrong with Pierre. I questioned Mom and she told me he was a mongoloid, medically known as Down syndrome. We did not know what this was all about. The entire family knew about Pierre but no one had told Henriette.

Since I lived two hours away it was a week or so before I got to see my godson, Pierre. I arrived at the Piché household to find that Pierre was sleeping. I asked if I could take a peek and maybe hold him. Henriette said, "Go ahead, he's such a good baby. He sleeps all the time and never cries." I picked him up from his sleep. He was so cute! I noticed that on one side of his face he had a droopy cheek. I teased and told Henriette this. She laughed and commented that one day both cheeks would look the same. Henriette at this point still didn't know that Pierre was Down syndrome and since I knew that he was, I examined him carefully and came to the conclusion that, yes, he did resemble a young girl in town that could pass for his sister and she was Down syndrome. Eventually the doctor in Gravelbourg told Henriette about Pierre.

Pierre has been a joy to all of us and has taught us a lot. He grew up with each of my children. They all seemed to know at a young age, two or three years old, that there was something different about Pierre. While visiting, they often asked why he didn't talk since he was older than they were. They enjoyed playing and sharing their toys and bicycles with Pierre.

Henriette and Gilles had a wall exhibiting pictures of their children's graduation pictures. Pierre's last year of school at Gravelbourg Elementary, in the Special Education Program, was 1987. I felt very strongly that Pierre should have a graduation picture on that wall, even if he could never graduate from grade 12. I decided to kidnap Pierre

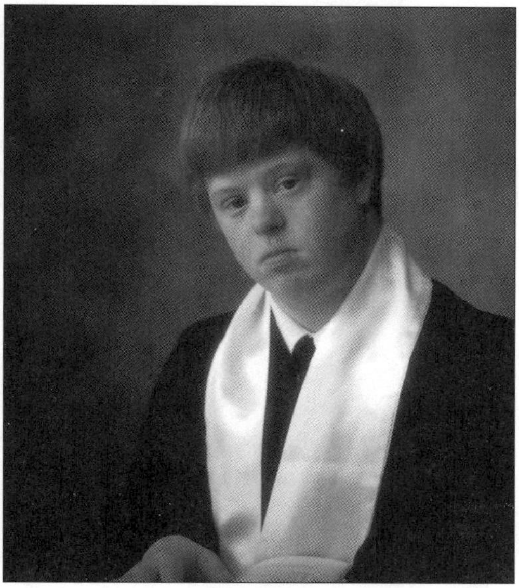

Graduation picture

from his class and with his teacher, Pat Prefontaine's permission, without Pierre's parents knowing about it, Mom and I took Pierre for the whole day to Assiniboia to a professional photographer and had his cap and gown picture taken. After receiving the photos, a few weeks later, I invited the Piché family for dinner, and Pierre, with a big smile, presented Gilles and Henriette his photos. They were so surprised and looked very pleased. It is with great satisfaction that I see his picture on the wall along with that of his siblings.

Pierre has many qualities. He is neat, organized and even though he doesn't speak very much he understands English and French. He often teases about his favourite snacks he is eating and not supposed to have like Coke, chips and popcorn. He loves any kind of sports and can't wait to help out at the farm.

If one is sad or hurting physically, he seems to feel it, and shows that he cares with a kiss, a pat on the back, or a hug.

Our whole family has been blessed, and lucky, to have Pierre as part of our family. He has made me a better person. Love you Pierre! XXX OOO

Camille Piché, ***Pierre's uncle***

A childhood memory I have is of Gilles and I, at a very young age, attending the public school at Gravelbourg, and Gilles, as we were walking back home, poking fun at a young boy who had Down syndrome. I remember feeling very sad for that boy who was different than the rest of us. I guess we just didn't understand.

My memory then takes me back to the time when Gilles and Henriette announced that their new-born son had Down syndrome; explaining how difficult it was for the doctor to tell them; the suggestion made that the child be placed in an institution; the heart-to-heart discussions that Gilles and Henriette had, resulting in keeping Pierre because "he is our son"; the tremendous efforts made to learn how to parent such a child and learn how to relate to him; the discovery of how special he and others like him are; the constant efforts made to have Pierre and his likes accepted in the community and their special needs provided for (family, acceptance, education, work, dignity, social life, etc . . .); organizing an association with parents, friends and community leaders to support mentally challenged people in Gravelbourg and surrounding communities; trying and trying, discarding false expectations and accepting performance limitations, rejoicing at every success, however minor. All the while love grew and deepened . . . ! Is it possible that this son would lead us in a very unconventional way, like another Special Son, to the heart of the Gospel, to unconditional love? How far we have come!

Desmond Hartney, *Pierre's cousin*

Pierre has a special relationship with young children. When I was born, Pierre was thirteen years old. I was quiet and I didn't cause much trouble so Pierre took a liking to me right away. There's a picture of Pierre and I, mounted on a wall at my home, with Pierre squeezing me tightly, as if he doesn't want to drop me. It was always comforting to be in the arms of Pierre.

As a child, going to Gravelbourg meant going to visit Pierre. When we would go to the swimming pool, everybody we met would say hi to Pierre. I'd think to myself, "Wow! This guy is cool!" When we got in the pool, there was no stopping Pierre. He would swim laps, jump off the diving board and even shoot some hoops. With his love for the water and his ability to swim under water with his eyes open, Pierre soon became known as "The Fish" to most of the family.

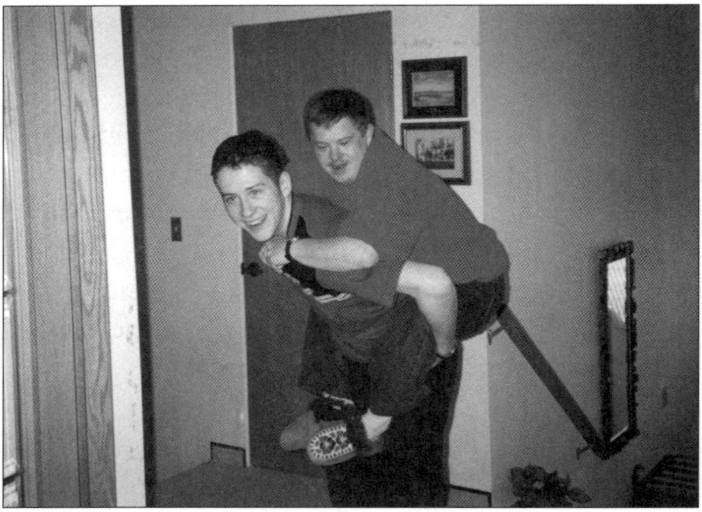

Getting ready for the wrestling match

The bond between Pierre and I grew stronger when we started wrestling. This tradition began one day in the basement of the Piché home. Pierre and I cleared the furniture from the middle of the room, squared off and began to wrestle. From that point on, whenever Pierre and I gather, we allocate some special time for our next bout. Even today, in my twenty-first year, the wrestling continues. Crowds of children (Kristyn, Monica, Loïc, Manoc and Chloé) assemble around us as we try to determine our next victor. The spectators chant out Pierre's name as he attempts move after move. The match goes back and forth, until Pierre seems to win for some unexplained reason. As I recover from the match, I think to myself, "Wow! This guy is cool."

1971–1982

First Teacher
Vera Silzer

I first became interested in special children by substitute teaching and helping in Assiniboia's Special Class. This wasn't entirely a new area to me as my oldest brother had Cerebral Palsey when he was born and was a T.M.R. person. In those days there was little help for him and I knew what it meant to grow up in a family with someone with such a handicap. I was so pleased to be able to work with these children. The summer before I started teaching the class I took a university class, one of many I took to help me teach and understand these children. I was so pleased to be given the opportunity to fill a dream of mine.

The fall of 1971 saw the opening of the class in Gravelbourg with seven children, including Pierre who was then only three years old, but came to school for one hour before Christmas and one-and-a-half after Christmas. You knew immediately upon meeting Pierre that he was loved and came from a loving home. His siblings loved him as much as any other and always looked out for him.

I always tried to do something with activity and something with listening and following orders. We would play games as Pierre loved activity even at that age. He liked to jump and run, play with the big ball. When we practiced for Special Olympics he was the happiest. He preferred that to reading and writing.

We worked a lot on life skills. You always had to put back what you took out and learn to handle all things with care. To wipe their own nose always was a challenge.

When Pierre was four and five he came to school for half days. This was quite an achievement for him but he grew to love it and always came in saying, "Hi." I would often get a hug as would the other children for they all just loved Pierre.

Pierre loved to perform whenever he had an audience and Special Olympics proved to be his time where he got lots of attention as he was so little and did so well. He won the hearts of many of the spectators.

Pierre, in spite of all the efforts, never learned to read other than to recognize his own name and a few other words. He knew where he lived and could walk to and from school by himself. He knew when someone was doing something they shouldn't be. He would shake his finger and say, "No." He knew how to dress himself, wash his hands; he did not like to be dirty.

Pierre had great difficulty holding pencils or crayons as his hands were very small and chubby. Thus we worked a lot on co-ordination and motor skills. He was always very proud of something he had accomplished and would show his Mom when she came for him and point to himself. Of course, his Mom was always pleased and would give him a hug. He would be so happy.

The years that I spent in Special Class will always hold a place in my heart. The parents were just A-One; they always were so co-operative and so good to me. I will always remember those years as the best years of my teaching experience. As a teacher you were appreciated by the parents and loved by all the children. What more could you wish for; every day was a blessing. I thank everyone who gave me the opportunity to grow and learn in this wonderful experience. I will remember it as a special part of my life.

1982–1987

Second Teacher
Pat Préfontaine

In September 1982, I was hired by the Gravelbourg School Division as the teacher for the Special Class. My professional passion over the years had been to work with students with special needs in different types of settings, but this assignment was a first. It was in a congregated classroom with a student enrollment of four. I was impressed with the dedication of the members on the division board and excited about the challenge of providing personal programs for each student.

The classroom had been in operation since 1971, with Vera Silzer as the teacher for the previous eleven years. Although I was a little apprehensive about taking over from someone who had fostered a working relationship with these students for such a long time, we got along fine as soon as I learned how to do things the "right way" (i.e., Silzer's). I was most fortunate because I had a class of students who were considerate, followed procedures, and were industrious.

Mornings were dedicated to the functional academics of language, reading, writing, and math. Afternoons were a little looser. The students each went to regular classrooms for inclusion right after lunch for a period. Then, we cranked up the music and did projects. I can still recall totally the words for 18-Wheeler by Alabama, and I get a giggle in my throat when I tune in CKRM radio.

Pierre participated in the morning activities patiently. We always discussed what each of us had done the evening before or what was going to happen at home that was exciting. On the days when I hadn't communicated with

Henriette and Gilles, I could always use the fall-back that Pierre was going to Mère's for chips and Coke after school. He acknowledged what we discussed by a "oui" (pronounced "way") or with "no-no-no" if he disagreed.

Pierre understood time by the activity, and he was never wrong, unless the hustle and bustle associated with the activity was out of schedule in his daily routine. For example, when we walked along one particular sidewalk and he saw the buses–he was gone: off to Mère's for chips. There were a few times, however, when we had to give chase because the bus had parked early to pick up students for a sports event.

Pierre communicated with a few key phrases, and as soon as you were smart enough to figure these out, things usually went along quite smoothly. When issues got a bit more complicated, he became a man of action. He would stand up, move his chair clear by giving it a push with his backside as he stood, straight and tall for a second, and then set off purposefully. It may be a quest for a pair of scissors, to get a kleenex, or to move someone out of his way.

If he felt I was expecting too much of him, he would stand up, walk over and put my arms by my side. He would then guide me over to my chair and sit me down. With a "yes" shake of his head, he would head back to his chair. A few minutes later, once I had given him his space, he would again stand up, come over, stroke my arm and help me back to his place. He would be ready to try again. Could he communicate! And he always did so with gentleness.

Pierre's favourite activity in school was to work on our projects. He particularly liked to do latch hook, making many rugs and cushion tops. His biggest pleasure was when he was finally able to take them home to Mamaman. I had to watch him towards the end of each job, however, because he would try to sneak them home before they were done!

He also liked to star in our Black Light presentations. For a few years, we put on productions for Christmas concerts and the Fashion Show. "Okay, P-Pat, if you want me to walk out there holding this piece of cardboard, I guess I can do it, but be aware that I may add my own flair to the performance." There were never any assurances that the performances would go off as planned.

We also completed a number of projects for Christmas so the students would have gifts for their parents and for the teachers and helpers in the school. I remember one Christmas when we were particularly pressed for time. I was rushing around the classroom providing support and encouraging them to work efficiently. Finally, I stopped and looked at them. They were all composed and relaxed. I was the only one who was flustered and in a panic. What a lesson I learned that day!

As Pierre reached puberty and had some personality alterations, he became less responsive. Although he participated less, I always felt he was aware of what we were doing and tried to comply once the expectations and the approach were adjusted.

Thanking you, Pierre, for teaching me so much. Thanks to you, I learned about patience, resilience, trust and devotion. It was an experience of a lifetime.

1987–2001

IPI–Workshop and Group Home
Rosemary Richmond, *Manager*

Pierre came into our lives on September 1, 1987, when he joined the work force at IPI as one of the founding participants. We had heard a lot about Pierre from his parents and Pat Préfontaine (his Special Ed teacher at the school). Henriette was concerned about Pierre making the adjustment to an entirely new situation. That morning, Pierre came into the Activity Centre with Henriette. She introduced him to the staff. Pierre gave us a small smile and shook our hands. He then proceeded on his own to go to each participant and introduce himself with a hand shake. So much for worrying about him making the adjustment; Pierre had made himself a part of the team.

In the early days of IPI, we learned about each other–our skills, interests and special abilities. His first jobs included making plastic wedding flowers, hooking rugs, macrameing hangers and doing various housekeeping duties. Pierre was the one who showed us how to make a flower bud and fluff it and the steps to hooking a rug. He was a very patient and gentlemanly teacher.

Pierre is a very dedicated worker who sticks with a task until it is completed. In his first year at IPI, Pierre would only stop working long enough for a quick drink or to eat lunch. He liked to work on only one project until it was completed (i.e. hook a rug until it was totally done) before he would change activities.

In 1990, Pierre moved into the group home. During his first year in the group home we saw many growths in Pierre. He became more aware of his surroundings and others, communicated more with words, interacted with his peers, initiated household chores and was more flexible in changing work duties or activities. Over the next three years, Pierre found his niche as a helper of other participants by assisting them with their lunch pails, pouring juice and generally watching out for them. Gradually, he began to learn to exercise his right to make choices and select activities. Instead of just doing activities set out for him, he began communicating to staff when he wanted to work at crushing cans or in the car wash.

Pierre has earned the respect and friendship of those around him with his kindness, gentleness and his commitment to his work and responsibilities. At each new stage of his life–joining the work force, moving out of the parental home, adjusting to new roommates and staff, facing the loss of family members, he has moved ahead with confidence and a positive attitude.

2001–

CORE
Judy Lancaster,
Team Leader, Programming

I know Pierre through the Day Program at CORE. I had seen him numerous times in the various work areas and he always struck me as a very shy man, who appeared to be overwhelmed at times by all the activities and commotion that was going on around him. I wasn't sure how he communicated, and from first glance I was not sure if Pierre had very much understanding about what was happening on a daily basis. He did not appear to show a lot of emotion and I always thought of Pierre as an individual who needed guidance for almost everything he did.

Some time later I was invited to a birthday party at the residence where Pierre lives. The party was for one of Pierre's roommates. The people had started arriving and Pierre was having a difficult time finding someone to assist him in following the routine he is familiar with. He appeared "lost" and continually kept looking out the window and at the door. He watched as people came into the room, his face never changing expression. He would look at the staff and then look at all the strangers as if trying to make sense of all the confusion.

I was sitting at the kitchen table talking to Pierre, trying to explain to him what was going on. I was asking him questions to which I was getting no response. All of a sudden, the door to the house opened and in walked Pierre's mother. I looked at Pierre and was about to tell him who had arrived and I saw Pierre look up and see his mother in the centre of the room. At this moment, this face that had just moments ago seemed to not be comprehending anything that was going on, absolutely lit up. Pierre looked at his mother with total adoration and love. He had a huge smile on his face and literally was glowing. I don't think I have ever seen so much love and emotion emit from someone's face as I did in that moment. Pierre and his mother moved towards each other and embraced. The moment was so spell binding I could not take my eyes off of them. The love between this mother and son was so moving it brought me to tears. In this single moment, I saw Pierre as a son, who was so devoted to his mother, that no matter what the handicap or barrier, shone through. Such utter devotion by both mother and child was something that I will never forget. Pierre instantly forgot all his fears or apprehensions, as the person that he most trusted and loved in the world, just by appearing, dissolved them all. Pierre now felt safe and secure, embraced in the most powerful emotion of love and in the total devotion that he felt for his mother. I don't think I will ever forget that look in his eyes, nor will I ever forget how this seemingly lost individual, was transformed in an instant, just by the presence of his mother.

Since that day I have seen this happen again and again with Pierre and his mother. This was not a one-time occurrence, but a lifetime of love that is between them. Pierre, even with his limitations, knows something that a lot of people strive for all their lives. That knowledge is love, from a parent who could have given up, or could have been discouraged, but went on to show her son what he meant to her. In return Pierre gives back the love unconditionally even though he is not able to use the spoken word, or buy her things, or tell others. Pierre's face spoke volumes that day, and made me realize that limitations placed on a person never diminish the capacity for feelings and emotions, and although Pierre is unable to communicate clearly, some expressions are there all the time, just waiting to be noticed and waiting for the right time to be shown. What a wonderful experience that was for me! I can only hope that my children look at me with half the love that Pierre showed his mother on that day.